The Cure for Good Intentions

A DOCTOR'S STORY

Sophie Harrison

FLEET
2022

FLEET

First published in Great Britain in 2021 by Fleet
This paperback edition published in 2022 by Fleet

1 3 5 7 9 10 8 6 4 2

A CIP catalogue record for this book is available from the British Library.

ISBN 978-0-349-14418-4

Typeset in Bembo by M Rules
Printed and bound in Great Britain by Clays Ltd, Elcograf S.p.A.

Papers used by Fleet are from well-managed forests and other responsible sources.

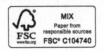

Fleet
An imprint of
Little, Brown Book Group
Carmelite House
50 Victoria Embankment
London EC4Y 0DZ

An Hachette UK Company
www.hachette.co.uk

www.littlebrown.co.uk

To Raj

This book is based on real events but I have changed anything and everything that might identify any of the people in it (other than my family, who appear as themselves).

When I was twenty-eight I left my job and went to train as a doctor. Amazing! people said, when I told them. Why are you doing that? I couldn't find a short answer. Sometimes I said, 'I had a revelation on a beach.' It was partly true.

I had been working as an editor for a publisher in London. I reorganised sentences and wrote comments in margins. 'Rephrase?' I wrote. 'Is this true?' In the manuscripts I read, the characters went places and did things. They rarely sat in offices. It was one of the things we editors had identified as lacking in contemporary fiction – realistic portrayals of employment. 'Why does no one write about work?' my colleague asked in a meeting one afternoon. The table was covered in coffee cups and the blind was down to stop a sunbeam that came in at certain times of year.

I loved my job. It was miraculous to be paid for reading books. But I was restless. I chewed biros until the plastic split. I skied my office chair from side to side: not all the way round – I wasn't a child. I went to the kitchen and boiled the kettle when no one wanted tea. I wandered round the office, visiting my colleagues at their desks.

Eventually I asked my boss for a sabbatical: I thought travelling might be a solution for restlessness. I applied for voluntary work and was accepted by a charity that sent people to teach English in Palestinian refugee camps across the Middle East.

The charity placed me in a camp in the south of Lebanon. I lived with two other volunteers in a bedroom in a Palestinian family's home. We arranged our sleeping mats against three of the walls.

We put a fan that we'd bought next to the fourth and adjusted it so it blew on each of us in turn. There was a pause while you waited for your gust. Sometimes I rolled onto the cold tiled floor. When it grew too hard I rolled back onto my mat. Our hosts did not have fans, and our arrival had deprived two sisters of their bedroom. They were now sharing with their grandmother; we could hear them bickering through the wall.

It was a Saturday night about three weeks into the trip. I had spent the morning cutting sixty clock faces out of cardboard in preparation for a lesson about telling the time. The clock faces were 'resources', a term we had learnt from one of the professional teachers volunteering alongside us. Resources were essential – the children paid attention to colouring, and lessons stalled without handouts – but I wished they didn't involve so much stapling. I didn't come to Lebanon to staple, I told my colleague. She showed me a dent that the scissors had made in her finger.

Now it was evening and a group of us had gone to the beach, where the children we taught never went. It wasn't a leisure beach – the sand was gritty and the sea was brown – but it was spacious after the camp, and there was a breeze. We drank a bottle of beer each and were immediately uplifted. I had a vision of a future in which I was truly useful. 'I'm going to go to medical school!' I announced. The other volunteers were supportive. It had become our default mode: encouragement was the main asset we had to donate. We punctuated our lessons with cries of 'Great!' and 'Fantastic!' while the children waited for us to calm down. 'Go for it!' everyone said to me now. 'Amazing!'

The applause obscured the impracticality. Why medicine, an expensive choice for which I was not obviously suited? I'd considered applying at school, but gave up as soon as I found science difficult. Now I was encouraged to think I'd had an epiphany.

The books I'd brought with me had given me ideas. One evening I read *Children of the Siege* by Pauline Cutting. Cutting had worked as a volunteer surgeon in a Palestinian camp near Beirut in the mid-1980s, while the camp was under siege from the Amal militia. The book opens with a boy called Bilal walking across an alley. 'High in a building outside the camp a sniper belonging to the Amal militia was watching the alleyway. When Bilal came into his sights he squeezed the trigger.' Bilal, 'a beautiful dark curly-haired boy of seven', is shot in the spine. Despite the medical team's attempts to help him, he is paralysed. Cutting worked in the camp for months, performing surgery in hopeless conditions.

Children of the Siege rendered the complexities of Palestinian-Lebanese history down to a furious list of atrocities and medicine's efforts to fix them. The simplicity was compelling. I felt I had always watched suffering from the sidelines, whereas Cutting and her colleagues had tried to make things better. I couldn't think of anything that I had made better.

The closest I'd been to pain had been illness in my family. When I was seven, J, my youngest brother, became sick. He was two. He hadn't been right for a while, my mother said afterwards. One January day she saw bruises and she took him to the doctor. At the end of school Mum wasn't there to collect me or my other brother, who was five. My father was waiting at the gate instead. Dad was holding his bike by the saddle: he could steer without using the handlebars, a skill I was keen to acquire. When we got home the house was empty.

J spent January, February and part of March in hospital with my mother. I wrote in my diary, 'J went to the doctor. Later he went to the hospital.' They admitted him to a ward and then to an isolation room. My father still went to work, but now he had to come home early to look after me and my brother, or we went to schoolfriends' houses until he was able to collect us.

J had been diagnosed with acute lymphocytic leukaemia, or ALL. In the 1950s, this was incurable. By the early 1980s the prognosis had just started to improve. The survival rate was still only forty per cent; there was mention of going to America for treatment. We didn't know any of this. Dad explained that J had something wrong with his blood, that there were white cells and red cells and that the white cells had gone mad. They were attacking the other cells and not working properly. He would have to stay in hospital and we would not be able to touch him or breathe on him in case he got a germ, which would be dangerous.

He could not leave his room. Sometimes we went to visit, although we couldn't see him unless Dad lifted us up, as his window was too high. We went to the hospital playroom and played with the toys that were meant for the sick children. Sometimes we lay on the floor of the corridor and talked to Mum and J through the grille in the bottom of the door.

At school the teachers spoke to us in soft voices, and one day I was allowed to use the scissors for the whole afternoon rather than having to pass them on when my time was up. This violation of the law of sharing gave me a bad feeling. I felt a pressure in my chest. At playtime I locked myself in the toilets. I stared at the paint on the door and tried to think of sad things to make myself cry: that our mother had left us, that my brother was ill. Eventually tears came, and then I couldn't stop them. Someone overheard and a teacher came and took me out to sit on a bench in the playground. I could see my friends watching us while they skipped.

I tried to be helpful at home. The parents at school had started a rota. Each day a different meal arrived at the gates or on the door-step, an ice-cream tub or a Pyrex dish with instructions Sellotaped to the lid. 'Two hundred degrees for twenty-five minutes,' I read to my dad. We put the meal in the oven. 'This isn't shepherd's pie!' my brother said. 'It is,' I replied. 'Shepherd's pie is different for different people.' At friends' houses, we ate delicious things we'd never had before, and other things we weren't sure about. Once someone's mother said, 'I don't expect you feel much like eating with what's going on,' and I agreed this was true, which it wasn't. We had just never had trifle before and were surprised by the wet cake.

We were in the middle of moving house when J got ill: my mother had broken off packing to take him to the doctor. The new house needed renovating, so my parents had rented a bungalow for us to live in while the builders worked. Moving day was the day after J went to hospital. I do not remember it at all, although I remember school was suddenly four fields rather than two streets away. The bungalow was cold. 'Outside walls,' Dad said. I hung over him as he tried to get the oven to turn on or the gas to ignite. I brushed my middle brother's hair and found him his teddy. His cheeks were red with eczema. I tucked dolls into cots and dead beetles into matchboxes.

J came home in March, although he went back in every day for another fortnight to have radiation treatment to his brain. He had a general anaesthetic each time to prevent him from moving during the treatment. Now he looked ill. He had no hair and was wearing a bobble hat even though it was spring. He didn't want to walk any more, although he was now three; he wobbled when he stood up. He also didn't want to eat. We had to sit with him until he had finished his plate. Mealtimes became very long. Sometimes my mother cooked liver. None of us liked it but we knew we had to eat it because it made your blood strong. Mum stood at the sink. While she had her back to us my middle brother and I helped J finish his plate. Liver tasted like iron, which was a strong metal, so we knew she was right.

The house was full of bobble hats and also knitted bees, which the neighbourhood had been making and selling in aid of a leukaemia charity. I was keen on these bees. They formed a significant secondary gain for me, along with the access to other families' biscuits and the syringes that a nurse had given us to play with. We didn't realise that in hospital syringes had needles attached and assumed we had been given functional equipment. We squirted pretend medicine into our teddies, and also into J when our mother wasn't looking.

Everything went back to a kind of normal except we now knew the word leukaemia, although I could not spell it. We knew there were diseases that could abduct you without warning. Across the fields near the bungalow you could just see the chimneys of the hospital. I asked Dad why they were so tall, and he explained it was because they needed big furnaces to burn all the hospital's dangerous waste, the poisons and blood and bacteria.

In the books I read I now recognised illness as a confirmation of reality. I looked to see if anyone could explain what it was for, or why it happened, or how to accommodate it into everyday life. Sometimes I was ill myself, with regular germs, and the sensations – bedtime in daytime, the rubber smell of the hot-water bottle, the dry taste of lemon barley water – got mixed up with what I was reading about and made it more real. When Peter Rabbit was put to bed with camomile tea, one tablespoonful to be taken at bedtime, I felt reassured by the similarities in our treatment. Even better was *Heidi*, in which Clara was raised from her wheelchair by fresh air and Swiss cheese; and *The Secret Garden*, in which Colin was cured by fresh air and digging. I liked a moral, and a cure. Aged ten, I read *What Katy Did*, in which Katy is punished for her impatient personality when she falls off a swing, injuring her back. She spends months in bed learning to endure. As soon as I'd finished it, I read it again, comforted by the conflation of sickness and health with rightful and wrongful behaviour. It confirmed that being helpful and good could stave off disaster. What useful things Katy learnt from her time in the School of Pain: about neatness, and staying cheerful; about stretching your forehead with your fingers so that lines wouldn't form. I was impressed by her tidy sick room. Rooms were important; they were always described in detail, the sick person's new whole world. We had never seen inside our brother's hospital room, except in glimpses through the window when Dad lifted us up and we saw a ball of blankets behind the bars of the cot, and our mother waving.

Medicine and doctors stayed in my head through school, even as I struggled with maths and science. At sixteen I sent off for a medical school prospectus. A catalogue arrived. I turned the pages and smelled the delicious smell, which was presumably magazine ink, although I thought of it as medical. I looked at the photographs. Students in a lab, holding pipettes. A student tilting her head at a patient, stethoscope resting on her blouse like a stole. None of it accessible without passing the science exams that I was failing. Chemistry contained an incredible unit of measurement called a mole, confusingly illustrated in my *Chemistry Made Easy* book by a cartoon mole. Every time I saw this black-and-white figure with his long nose and whiskers, I thought of the cartoon gerund drawn by Ronald Searle in the fictional schoolboy's autobiography *The Compleet Molesworth*. The gerund, a round animal with a long proboscis, sits by itself, a tear on his cheek. 'A gerund shut out. No place for it in one of my sentences.'

There was no whimsy in chemistry. 'It's not difficult if you concentrate,' said the teacher as I stared at Avogadro's constant,

$6.02214086 \times 10^{23}$ mol^{-1}. It became clear I could not concentrate. English was an easier subject, in which you read books and said what you thought they were about. Daydreaming was acceptable, because that was thinking, and it was fine to be uncertain about facts, because that was questioning. Science was unimpressed by ambivalence, a word I used in every English essay.

After graduating from my English degree, I worked as a waitress. At one job the manager asked me to water the plants that stood on the windowsills. I went round with a watering can, looking out of the windows as I poured. The staff were laughing. 'They're plastic,' said the bus boy when I'd finished. I got a job writing software manuals, and then TV listings. 'The TV listings are the most-read page in the newspaper,' my boss said. 'Except for the crossword. There is no margin for error. One mistake and we get a thousand complaints. It's life-or-death stuff.'

One day I went for an interview for a sales job at a publisher. They turned me down. A month later I got a letter from the same publisher. I was living in a flat in London at the time. All the post for the building landed on the communal doormat, where it lay until someone picked it up. There was a shoe print on the envelope, but it couldn't spoil the fact that this was a good-looking envelope made from heavy cream paper. The letter inside said a job had come up as an editorial assistant. I felt as elated as I did on the beach six years later.

I had no more thoughts about medicine until I went to the camp. On the first day there I discovered one of the other volunteers was a medical student. She didn't seem to think this was interesting or unusual. It was as though she had stepped out of my old prospectus; she had even brought her stethoscope with her. I hassled her with questions about mending the injured and healing the sick. But she wanted to talk about politics.

The father of the family we were staying with had been having pains in his chest, and his daughter took him to a clinic in the town. The visit was expensive, and everyone in the house was keyed up with anticipation. As he stood in the hall waiting to leave, the women pressed items on to their father – a scarf, a handkerchief, a packet of food. But the trip was an anti-climax; the appointment lasted ten minutes, and the doctor spoke too fast. The heart was not right, but it wasn't clear in what way. The daughter came to find the medical student to see if she could help. The daughter took a roll of paper out of her handbag, and the student smoothed it out. The old man came to watch. The student ran her finger under the zigzag of the ECG. 'They're just ectopic beats,' she said to the daughter. 'Common, not harmful. Don't worry.'

Once again medicine was confirmed as useful. The student had dispensed with ambivalence and identified the facts. She could have assisted Pauline Cutting. Whereas I had taught my class of teenage girls Keats's 'Ode to a Nightingale'.

I came home ready for medical school. On the beach it had seemed a simple matter of enthusiasm. Back in Britain the obstacles were obvious. I didn't have the right qualifications, except for an A level in biology. I didn't have any experience. The medical student had laughed at my adulation; now I realised she was also laughing at my naivety.

I began volunteering at a hospice for patients with advanced Aids, once a week, after work. I had no idea what I was doing there. 'Just sit with them, it reminds them the outside world exists,' said the nurse supervisor. I sat in the lounge with the patients and watched television. I had an unread manuscript in my bag, but I didn't get it out in case I had to explain who I was. Everybody smoked, as did I; I lent out my lighter. Was this useful? The virus, untreated, had contributed to the patients developing brain damage, by a mechanism that I didn't understand. We were all working hard to get lung cancer. Every week, a patient called Smith and I discussed his main interest, the Billboard Top One Hundred Songs of 1999. 'Ask me what was Number Five,' he said. I didn't know. 'Yes, that's right, Number Five was indeed the immortal "... Baby One More Time"!' He yelled the first line of the song. The others complained that they couldn't hear the television. On Valentine's Day I bought Smith a card and some chocolate. I picked the least loving card I could find, not wanting to be inappropriate. He wanted cigarettes, but that didn't seem the right gift, medically.

I had met a medical student and I had learnt that untreated Aids could cause dementia. I knew this wasn't enough for a successful medical school interview. But I didn't know any doctors; there were none in my family, and I hadn't come across any during my English degree, or at work. At last my brother arranged for me to spend an evening in a hospital shadowing one of his friends, who was a junior doctor. I met the doctor at seven, at the start of his shift. His bleep went off immediately, and every few minutes it bleeped again. There was a phone halfway down each corridor, where he would stop to reply to his bleep while I stood watching him use the phone. 'I have no idea why you're choosing to do this,' he said. At midnight I went home. It seemed very late; the street was empty, the air cold and fresh. The doctor still had nine hours of his shift left. 'Tip for your interview?' he said. 'They will ask you, "Why do you want to be a doctor?" Do not say, "Because I want to help people." Everyone says that.'

I arranged another shadowing session, in A&E. I hung around the department until a consultant saw me sitting on a chair and took me to see a patient. She was a beautiful young woman, exactly my idea of an emergency patient. She had run into a glass door and cut a flap of skin from her arm.

The consultant asked the patient to turn her head away. He had a warm voice, as befitted this scene from *ER*. I stood next to him, holding the injured arm under a sterile piece of paper while he sutured. 'If you take the stitches out early enough you don't get the little dots along the sides of the scars, just the scars,' said Dr Smith. There was dried blood in stripes on the patient's hands and feet. 'It looks like a horror film,' she said. The consultant said he hated horror films: 'I can't bear blood.' 'Is that a joke?' she said.

The suturing took a long time. Dr Smith and I chatted. He wanted to talk about books, about a novel he'd read about a surgeon. 'Mind-blowing,' he said. I couldn't believe I was in a hospital and talking about literature with a doctor. This was it. I thought the book he was talking about was terrible, but I didn't want to spoil the moment by saying so. Meanwhile, every book I read about medicine further decreased my confidence.

I read *A Country Doctor's Notebook*, Mikhail Bulgakov's semi-autobiographical stories about his experiences as a newly qualified doctor posted to a remote Russian province in the 1920s. It made me anxious. I did not think I would ever be able to diagnose a syphilis outbreak or bluff my way through an obstructed labour. Bulgakov's doctor worries too: how can he do this nerve-racking thing, he's never done it before, it's impossible, says his protagonist, before immediately getting on with the task at hand. He saves a child from diphtheria by inserting a steel tube into her throat. He amputates a young woman's leg.

After reading *Cancer Ward* by Solzhenitsyn and half of *The Magic Mountain* by Thomas Mann, I looked for something lighter.

'Ooh Dr Finlay!' someone said when I told them I wanted to go to medical school. I immediately started watching *Dr Finlay's Casebook*, a 1960s *Doc Martin*, one moral per episode. A. J. Cronin, the creator, was a doctor who also wrote nineteen novels, including

The Citadel ('a moving story of tragedy, triumph and redemption').
There was a good chance I would read all nineteen: tragedy, triumph and redemption were what I was after. I watched the film of his novel *The Stars Look Down*, scrutinising it for medical information. Released in 1940, it is the story of Davey Fenwick, played by Michael Redgrave, a working-class boy from a mining village. In an early scene Davey is writing, bent over a lamplit desk, the eternal image of a medical student. In fact, he goes on to become a teacher. Ma Fenwick is unimpressed. 'You and your fancy scholarships,' she says. Davey's father has a cough. 'This cough will never kill me, Davey,' he promises. It doesn't. The grasping mine owner sends the men down the mine and it collapses. Some of the victims are brought to the surface. There is a close-up of a ventilator being used on one of the men: it looks like a pair of bellows. A doctor appears to treat another of the victims with Swedish massage. Davey's father is trapped underground. He sustains one of the lads with cough drops, his motif throughout.

Cronin's stories had everything I loved about medicine in fiction. Medicine created drama, and the opportunity to experience emotion without yourself coming to harm. When someone got sick or was injured you knew what you were supposed to feel. If they worsened and died, or were healed and saved, you felt sadness, or relief. The accident or the illness and the emotions it generated gave time a form. Life no longer flowed past, a stream of this and then that, with no clear indication of what anything meant. Instead there was fear, dread, suspense. A structure; and a moral guide from that.

I signed up for an evening class in A-level chemistry at an adult education college near my flat. The students sat without whispering or doodling, aware this was a second chance. We never acknowledged each other. Our eyes were fixed on the whiteboard where the lecturer was drawing carbon molecules. Occasionally someone asked a question, and everyone listened to the answer and wrote down what the teacher said. Occasionally the teacher made a joke, but he stopped after a few weeks of teaching our class.

At the same time I signed up for an exam called the GAMSAT, which would allow me to apply to the graduate entry to medicine courses. There were no evening classes for the GAMSAT. I tried to teach myself using past papers. I sent off money, and an A4 envelope came in the post. When I read the papers, I was confounded.

> 12) A person stands on a scale in an elevator. He notices that the scale reading is lower than his usual weight. Which of the following could possibly describe the motion of the elevator?
>
>   A. It is moving down and slowing down.
>   B. It is moving down at constant speed.
>   C. It is moving up and slowing down.
>   D. It is moving up with constant speed.

I read the online forums about the exam. It is a test of stamina, they said. It is a test of self-belief. Do not engage with the questions. Do not picture things in your mind: extract the meaning and solve them.

I got a borderline pass on the GAMSAT and an AS level in chemistry. Two medical schools offered me interviews – one in London, and one in a different city. The London interview took place first. 'Why do you want to do medicine?' the panel asked. I couldn't help it: I wanted to help people. There were three interviewers, taking it in turns to ask questions. 'A lot of people say that,' the woman in the middle said. 'Do you want to add anything else?' My brain filled with romance. An ECG in Lebanon; the taste of a cough sweet as I lay in bed reading *By the Shores of Silver Lake*: 'The fever had settled in Mary's eyes and Mary was blind.' Keats, a trainee surgeon before he became a poet, extracting a bullet from a woman's neck. I mentioned scientific curiosity and how does untreated Aids cause dementia? My application was rejected.

The other medical school gave me a place. The school was brand new; it was still being built when I went for an interview. It encouraged students from 'non-traditional' backgrounds. There was nothing non-traditional about my background, but my age and my English degree counted as untypical. They took many applicants from the Access to Medicine course (an alternative to A levels for older students), and over a third of us were 'mature', ranging in age from twenty-one to forty-two.

On the first day I took a bus to the campus. I walked up the steps of the new building. The windows of the canteen were decorated with a decal of an ECG trace. I had rented a room in a flatshare and put a lamp on my desk. It was all coming together.

I had a new book in my bag, *The Oxford Handbook of Clinical Medicine*, which the students called the 'Cheese and Onion' after its yellow and green cover. The cover was plastic, like no book I had owned before – built for a life of action and bloodstains. I thought of it as the Book of Everything. How to examine a hand, an eye, a heart. How to put in a cannula. How to take blood. When Tony Hope and Murray Longmore put the first edition together they wrote it out in longhand on squared paper so as to be sure they could fit everything in. Each double-page spread took one subject – abnormal heart rhythms, asthma – and gave you the facts.

The Cheese and Onion is essential, a lecturer said on the first day, holding the book up to show us. I stopped myself waving my copy back at him. After lectures, I went to the canteen and got out my notebook. I flicked through the handbook. Here was Barthel's

'Index of Activities of Daily Living', a scoring system for degrees of infirmity. You could add up the numbers under each heading to score the level of your disability in a particular field, e.g.:

<u>Feeding</u>
    0 Unable
    1 Needs help in cutting, spreading butter, etc.
    2 Independent (food provided within reach)

I marvelled at the specificity of 'food provided within reach'. Underneath the index were some words about independence and interdependence, and then a quote from John Donne. 'No man is an Island, intire of it selfe.' I had not expected to find a metaphysical poet here, next to a numerical system for assessing bowel control.

As I'd looked up illnesses, I'd felt my ignorance grow thicker. I had found the pages on ALL and felt ashamed I'd only ever called it leukaemia. I hadn't known there were several different kinds. 'Aim to tailor therapy to the exact gene defect, and according to individual metabolism. Monoclonal antibodies, gene-targeted retinoids, cytokines, vaccines, and T-cell infusions are relevant here.' Of these, I knew what a vaccine was, though I couldn't see the relevance. I reconstructed the treatment as understood by an eight-year-old. I remembered drips (difficult to extricate from the idea of a dripping tap); radiotherapy (filed in my mind alongside Marie Curie and nuclear war); and chemotherapy (handfuls of tablets next to uneaten plates of food). I looked up lumbar punctures; the diagram made me nauseous. I still didn't understand the rationale for radiotherapy. 'He didn't like being pinned down,' Mum told me years afterwards. How had I not seen his suffering, or my parents' suffering either? I'd thought only about myself: what was for pudding, if there'd be custard, if anyone at school had seen me crying and how I could persuade them that they hadn't.

After several years of treatment J was declared better, and once he was five years from diagnosis without relapsing we could say he was cured. His illness had reached a conclusion, if you overlooked repercussions and after-effects. I never met his doctors or his nurses, although I'd seen a person in a mask and gown bending over his bed. People wearing stethoscopes had passed us in the corridor. Once a man in a white coat told us not to lie on the floor.

In my new room I kept the *Oxford Handbook* on my desk. I sometimes read it by the light of my lamp, like a fictional medical student. I liked the quotation on the title page. It was by William Osler, the Canadian physician who invented bedside teaching. I didn't know if he'd said it or written it. I pictured him bedside, as he'd invented the concept, the patient under a tight white sheet, Osler speaking from under his nineteenth-century moustache.

He who studies medicine without books sails an uncharted sea, but he who studies medicine without patients does not go to sea at all.

Hospital

Throughout medical school doctors asked us what we were going to do, or what we were going to be. I thought it was obvious that we were going to be doctors. I hadn't understood how many kinds of doctor there were: gastroenterologists, nephrologists, paediatricians, anaesthetists, pathologists, radiologists. A different surgeon for each body part. A paediatrician couldn't operate and a stroke physician couldn't deliver babies. With this realisation, each hospital placement acquired a new intensity. Now it was a search for what one of the students called his forever organ. On the respiratory ward I imagined a life of lungs. On hepatology, livers. The doctors shared ancient stereotypes to help us decide. Neurologists brainy; pathologists chilly. 'What is the difference between God and an orthopaedic surgeon?' an orthopaedic surgeon asked us. We knew the answer, but we didn't like to say. 'God doesn't think he's an orthopaedic surgeon.'

There was also general practice, which took place outside the hospital, in the normal world, which was now an environment called the community. The community wasn't mentioned much in hospital, where most of my training took place. We knew patients came from there and had to be returned there; otherwise we didn't think much about it. We forgot that we lived there ourselves. This was fair enough, as for periods of time we didn't. In one residential hospital placement, the sheets on my bed had PROPERTY OF SMITH HOSPITAL TRUST printed on them, and for that placement I belonged to Smith Hospital Trust too.

We did hear from GPs occasionally, as they phoned the hospital doctors to request admission for one of their patients. 'Yes?' the registrar said. A noise went into her ear. She wrote the details on a piece of paper. 'Fine,' she said. The hospital doctors dispensed with introductions or salutations; the prevailing style was clipped. I understood this to mean that they were busy. Later, the patient would arrive at A&E or the Acute Admissions Unit, sometimes escorted by a partner or a friend, always with the same look of baffled excitement. He held a letter from the GP in his hand like a ticket and from the moment of his arrival he tried to give it to someone – the desk clerk, the clinical support worker, the triage nurse. No one wanted it. At last a junior doctor came and opened the envelope, but he only glanced at the letter. 'We need to start from the beginning in here,' the doctor said.

My first training hospital was a big Victorian building, once the city's workhouse, which had been extended as the population grew. Extra buildings, including a tower block, had been stuck on as they were needed. As in all British hospitals, the entrances and corridors were layered with signs. Arrows pointed in every direction: some appeared to indicate the ceiling. At a different hospital, later in my training, a registrar summarised religious belief by gesturing at the UP and DOWN arrows next to the lift. 'Believer ... non-believer,' he said. The morgue was in the basement. That hospital had been built on a hill. The third floor in the lower buildings was the ground floor in the higher ones. Every visitor was lost.

A few years into my training I was used to hospitals. I no longer registered the scuffed pastel walls or the contradictory signage or the notices explaining Six Steps to Washing Your Hands. But at the start I noticed everything. On the second day of my first placement, a patient I had been sent to talk to began to cough. It was nothing spectacular, just a soft 'hem hem' sound. Then he opened his mouth and blood came out. It ran down his chin, over his chest, and made a puddle on his blanket. I stared at him. He waved his hands at me and tried to speak. Bubbles formed and popped on his lips. The patient in the next bed pressed the buzzer for the nurse. That night in bed I remembered the blood. I had tasted blood in my own mouth only when my first teeth fell out. A metal taste. I thought of liver. The patient's blood had turned black as it soaked into the green blanket. Haemorrhage. 'An escape of blood from a ruptured vessel,' I googled.

The next day we were back in lectures. A slide went up, a photograph of someone's leg. It was flushed red from ankle to knee. 'Dolor ... rubor ... calor ... tumor,' said the lecturer, the Latin names for the four signs of inflammation (pain, redness, heat, swelling). My neighbour had drawn a leg in her notebook and was cross-hatching it in red biro. 'Cellulitis is an infection of the skin's deepest layer: does anyone know what that's called?' the lecturer asked. The front row raised their hands. My neighbour added a shoe and started colouring it in.

Each dusk, after the fluorescent lights of the hospital, the streetlights seemed dim. The passengers on the bus seemed naive. I felt I'd seen how things really were. It reminded me of Frank Netter's anatomy watercolours: I had a set of his flashcards back at the room I was renting. When Netter wants to illustrate some deep-lying organ, he adds a little tool that holds the layers of skin and muscle out of the way like a curtain tie-back. After a day in the hospital it was difficult to close the curtain again, to forget what could go wrong with your lungs, your liver, your blood, your kidneys, your brain.

As a medical student and then as a new doctor, I learnt by observation. Other doctors, and nurses, told me what to do, or I watched them and copied them. I copied so thoroughly that I ended up absorbing other people's sentences, so that one day I heard myself saying 'hear hooves, think horses' to a colleague, to encourage him to prioritise a commonplace diagnosis over anything more exotic (do not go straight to zebras). Every doctor in Britain uses this analogy.

The hospitals loved hierarchy. Everyone was 'junior' or 'senior'. 'Ask your senior,' the nurses said. 'Has your senior had a go?' the anaesthetics F2 said when you bleeped her to ask for help with a cannula. We arranged ourselves in ranks. At the bottom the medical students, not yet qualified, nor paid. Then the F1s, Foundation Year Ones – previously called house officers – in their first year of work; the F2s, in their second, formerly SHOs or senior house officers; the registrars, who might be one year or ten years into their specialist training; and finally the consultants. The system flattened the differences between us. All we did was work, with short hiatuses for limited and predictable leisure activities. We liked the same television programmes and holidayed in the same places and aspired to the same cars, although there was always some junior doctor in the news winning *MasterChef* or scaling Mount Kenya to make the rest of us feel inadequate. We spoke the same language, but we differed in how we touched our patients – in what order we patted them down, whether we gripped Mr Smith's shoulder or preferred to hover just out of his reach.

The first few months of hospital took place in a foreign language. 'He's gone for an oesophagoduodenoscopy,' I told the consultant, finding a bed empty during the ward round. 'Sweetie,' said the registrar, 'you can just say "OGD".' The acronyms didn't follow any rules. Sometimes you said the letters – 'TIA' instead of 'transient ischaemic attack'; always 'MI', never 'myocardial infarct'. But sometimes you pronounced the acronym as if it were a word. 'Stemmy', which was STEMI, and 'enstemmy' (NSTEMI): two different kinds of heart attacks. The elderly fractured their 'nofs' (the neck of the femur: that is, they had broken their hips). To the orthopaedic surgeons, they *were* nofs – 'We're expecting the nof, when is she coming down?' 'We need to get salt,' the doctors said (speech and language therapy). Sometimes the tangle happened the other way round. In a clinic, the consultant had me read out the GP's referral letters to him before I called the patient. 'He is allergic to pollen, house dust and ee-dot-gee-dot-gee-dot,' I read. What was this acronym? The consultant was gentle enough that I dared a question. 'What's ee-gee-gee?' 'Comes out of a chicken,' he replied.

Along with terminology came the hospital style. We discussed the patient as if he were a piece of machinery, a car or a plane, in need of support and servicing. We prescribed 'maintenance fluids'. If you gave a medicine, you could say that the patient had morphine or adrenaline 'on board'. We might say a dehydrated patient was 'running very dry'. Wetness and dryness were preoccupations. At handover, the exiting doctor would relay a paragraph of medical terminology about a patient and conclude 'he's as dry as a crisp'. Crispiness was a common problem, usually caused by something we'd done – making the patient nil by mouth, or failing to give him enough intravenous fluids. However, 'wetness' was also to be avoided, and it was best not to 'over-fill' elderly patients by prescribing multiple bags of normal saline or running fluids through the IV too fast.

Where an astronaut might say 'it's not brain surgery', we would say 'it's not rocket science'. All unnecessarily elaborate blood test results were described as 'serum rhubarb' and all elderly ladies were called 'old dears'. Any obvious diagnosis had to be described as 'barn door'. You also had to give all patients a cockney accent when telling any medical anecdote. 'So he says, "Doc, is it me 'art?"' etc. In anecdotes told by doctors the patient always addressed the doctor as 'Doctor' or 'Doc'. At work, only the Filipino nurses did this, and they sounded ironic.

We spoke to patients in what we believed to be everyday speech, although it was in fact another language again: infantile, nursery-inflected. We called abdomens 'tummies' and warned 'this might feel a bit chilly'. We used soothing, neutered verbs. I learnt to ask patients to 'pop' off their clothes before 'hopping' up onto the bed, where I would just 'slip' this nameless thing I was holding up their noses or down their throats or up their 'tail end'. Along with all the popping, I sometimes suggested a 'quick feel' of the tummy or the wrist (we stopped sniggering after a few months, and a few months after that forgot it was funny). Sometimes we preferred a 'quick look'. There was a variety of equipment, but all of it was special. We sent patients for a 'special scan' or a 'special test', or arranged for them to be examined using a 'special camera'. If we found they needed it, they were fitted with a pacemaker – 'a special device to help regulate your heartbeat' – or arranged for repair of their hernias using a 'special kind of mesh'. Although it was all special, I also told people 'we do this all the time'. Sometimes I alerted the patient that 'this might be uncomfortable'. Before I stuck needles into people's bodies I gave a warning I'd learnt from listening to other people giving warnings: 'sharp scratch!' or 'bee sting!'

We students were sent on ward rounds to expand our learning.

Two or three of us would trail after the consultant. We carried our coats and our bags with us, as there is a shortage of storage space in British hospitals (and thieves). Our luggage increased our awkward and temporary air. Some rounds involved large groups of people. Alongside the doctors and nurses, you might get the physiotherapist or the occupational therapist or the pharmacist, or – in one hospital – the cleaner, an elderly Pakistani man who had learnt medicine though spending so much time on the wards. When we arrived at a patient's bed he would be there before us, dusting the curtain rail or mopping under a chair. He would hover among the doctors, pulling out the notes from the trolley and diving for the observations chart, which he would hold so you could transcribe the numbers. After the round moved on he would take you aside for a debrief: 'Did you get *full* tuberculosis history?'

Sometimes the consultant noticed us. 'Where are the students?' she said. 'You – in the cardigan – why are you carrying your coat? Are you planning on leaving us? Come here and examine this patient's chest and tell me what you find.' The patient had either been handled by many previous students, in which case he knew more than you (some patients whispered tips – 'It's a thoracotomy scar!'), or he would be straining to catch everything you said, hoping for an insight into his illness. We were not reassuring. As medical students we preferred the rare and terrible diagnoses – the zebras – over common, treatable illnesses – the horses. When nervous or excited we tended to issue lists: 'Something malignant? Invasion of the brachial plexus? Horner's syndrome?'

When the hospital was full, which was often, teaching rounds became 'business' rounds, with no time for a lecture on the classical signs of liver failure. A business round for a medical 'firm', or team, could take half a day or longer. We stood by a bed; walked to the next bed; stood by a bed again. There might be forty or fifty patients to see. It was hard work without involving any actual work for us. The F2s and registrars huddled to exchange information. I looked at the patients in their beds, but I didn't stare. If someone was wearing a bandage or had a disfigurement, I particularly didn't look at that, so that I didn't seem to be gawping. I studied the things on the patients' bedside tables instead – their books, their magazines, their sweets. The magazines were full of medical drama: catastrophic accidents, incredible injuries. Sometimes I wished I was in the bed instead of the patient, wrapped in a blanket, sucking a lemon sherbet, reading 'My Baby was Born with Three Legs'.

As a junior doctor I remained a trainee, although I was also working, and getting paid. Now we were meant to learn on the job. Formal teaching dwindled to an hour a week. We would assemble in a side office off the ward, and the consultant or one of the registrars would give us some teaching. They sometimes overlooked the ignorance of their juniors. Once an orthopaedic registrar showed us forty numbered slides of different eponymous fractures. Salter-Harris I, Salter-Harris II, Galeazzi, Monteggia, reverse Barton. At 20/40 someone whispered 'Half time!' 'I didn't know we *had* that many bones,' one of the F1s said. Some sessions were 'self-directed', which meant teaching each other. We copied websites into PowerPoint and then gave a presentation, newly expert on epilepsy or ovarian cysts. 'Here I have summarised my knowledge of bacterial vaginosis,' said my colleague, clicking to a blank slide.

Starting work as an F1, the most junior junior on the rounds, I came to understand why the seniors had not had time to teach us anything. The juniors came in early and left late. We had to record our hours in a diary, for European Working Time monitoring, but it was better not to put them down correctly, as to write down your actual hours brought you compulsory attendance at seminars with titles like 'Better Time Management for Failing Doctors', where a lecturer of unknown provenance would show us a PowerPoint about 'The Five Types of Inefficient Doctor' and ask us to ensure we emptied our stress buckets every day.

On one surgical team, the F1s arrived at five in the morning to give themselves enough time to get everything 'buffed' before the round started at 7.30. First you made a list of your firm's patients and where they all were. This depended on how busy the previous day's 'take' had been – how many new patients had been admitted. Every hospital had a dream. In this dream, surgical patients were admitted to surgical wards, elderly patients to care of the elderly wards, and respiratory patients to respiratory wards. In real life, once wards ran out of space, new patients were sent wherever there was a bed. We feared losing these patients, the 'outliers', as they languished on a distant ward, tended by nurses skilled in the wrong specialty, forgotten by the ward round who weren't expecting to go to gynaecology to see their patient with liver disease.

At last the consultant or the registrar would arrive. 'Shall we?' As F1, you pushed the notes trolley. You had to find the right ward and the right bed, check you had the right patient, extract the correct file from the trolley and find the first blank page in the notes without detaching all the other pages from their treasury tags and showering them across the floor. 'Like a buffoon,' as my F2 described it. 'Don't be a buffoon.'

As the consultant or registrar talked, we documented everything in the notes. We wrote the Hx:/ or history, an Ex:/ or examination, the Obs:/ or observations, and the P:/, which was the plan. The P was the only part anyone cared about, because it told everyone what was meant to happen next – perhaps some more blood tests, or an X-ray, or 'mobilise' – the clinical term for getting out of bed.

Or – the grail – 'MEDICALLY FIT FOR DISCHARGE'. One care of the elderly firm I worked for had had a rubber stamp made with this diagnosis, which we would stamp into the notes after writing the Hx and Ex and Obs. For some patients we stamped daily. Monday: MEDICALLY FIT. Tuesday: MEDICALLY FIT. Wednesday: MEDICALLY FIT. But the patient remained in hospital, with nowhere safe to be discharged to, no 'care package' available for home, and no space at, or finances for, a nursing home. The occupational therapists and the physiotherapists worked on getting their patients to mobilise. They took them to the ward kitchen to test their ability to operate the microwave or make a cup of tea. Every stairwell contained an elderly person proving themselves on the stairs. The therapists also visited patients' homes to ensure they were fit for re-occupation. This was how the OT found Mr Smith's budgies: they flew up in a yellow cloud when she opened his front door. At night they were roosting on his shower rail. 'Bath full of bird crap, absolutely plastered in it,' she said as I stamped the notes like a librarian. MEDICALLY FIT FOR DISCHARGE. Eventually Mr Smith fell ill again, with an infection caught on the ward, and we retired the stamp and went back to writing the original P: 'Antibiotics. Mobilise.'

It was halfway through a night at that hospital that my key card stopped working, trapping me in a long corridor that bridged two different sites. Unlike the wards, it was cold. After swiping the card through the reader a few times, I gave up. I wished it was a key-coded door, because you could always find the code written somewhere, if you searched the wall and the frame for long enough. (Sometimes you found it right above the keypad, perhaps written by the same person who had stuck a Post-it note with the computer password to a computer in the doctors' office.) I peered through the locked door, tapping the window. Soon there was a jingle behind me: it was the night security guard, hung about with keys, phones and ID badges. 'You rattle, don't you?' I said as he opened the door. 'It's a deliberate strategy,' he said. 'Let them hear you coming, gives them time to run.'

A few weeks later I attended a talk about improving efficiency in hospital. It was in the doctors' office on the ward, a cupboard containing three old computers, one of which everyone avoided as the M and I keys no longer worked ('I just write "heart attack",' said the F1). The talk was illustrated with clip-art diagrams about a Japanese car manufacturer – I think it was Honda. In the pictures, Honda cars slid through Honda's flawless systems to emerge shining and on schedule. The speaker was fired up with how wonderful the world could be; his eyes were bright. On the window ledge behind him was the usual doctors' litter – an empty pizza box, a squeezed Capri-Sun packet and a box of expired blood bottles. Dirty coffee cups stood on every surface. I pictured Honda's chief executive taking it all in, before making the Japanese gesture for 'burn it all to the ground and start again'.

Surgical rounds started earliest and moved fastest, as the surgeons raced to get to theatre; their interest dwindled the further post-operative the patients became, as the number of inpatient days post-op can correlate with complication ('Why is he still here?' one consultant asked about any patient admitted for longer than three days. 'Never say: "because you ballsed up his op",' the F1 said later.) The weekend orthopaedic ward round was dreaded. All the surgeons wanted was to get to theatre so that they could start the list and get through that day's operations. A cancellation meant starving an elderly person for a day, only for her hip to remain broken at the end of it. But they had to round every post-operative patient before they could go down, and there had been three full teams operating the day before. It seemed like hundreds of patients, and each one was a fractured (#) nof, distinguished only by being a LEFT or a RIGHT. We ran from bed to bed, condensing every entry to the classical surgical trio of

Hx: #NOF.
Ex: Obs stable. Afebrile.
P: Continue.

One Saturday I wrote this in the notes of an elderly woman whose fractured hip had been successfully fixed the previous day. I opened her chart to make sure that the observations were indeed stable. The round had moved on. This habit of checking was making me fall behind. As the most junior that day, I should have been first to each bed, ready with a concise summary for my seniors ('Four words would be best,' the F2 advised. 'Medically fit for discharge'). The registrar had already told me off for writing too slowly and had asked if I was dyslexic.

The patient's blood pressure was documented as 80/40. Her pulse wasn't recorded. I felt apprehensive as I went to shake her by the shoulder. She didn't wake up. Fuck, I thought. 'Mr Smith,' I called to the consultant; the round turned to look at me. 'This lady is unresponsive.'

'Fucking HELL,' said Mr Smith. I didn't know if he was angry that she had died or angry that I'd checked. I could feel his thoughts travelling down to theatres: the staff fidgeting, the anaesthetists looking at the clock, the nurses apologising to the patients and their families.

One of the nurses ran to phone 2222, the universal number for the arrest team in British hospitals. Someone went to get the arrest trolley. I tipped the patient's head into the head tilt-chin lift position to make sure her airway was open. I looked at her chest to see if she was breathing and listened at her mouth, and at the same time put my fingers on her neck to see if I could feel a pulse at the carotid artery. These are the first steps of the Resuscitation Council UK algorithm, the standard in every British hospital. The algorithm is inflexible. Whether the patient has had a heart attack, a stroke, or has drowned, whether he is lying in a puddle of blood, faeces, water, or in his bed, you follow the same steps in the same order. There is no scope for creativity or improvisation. It is a tool designed to achieve the best possible chance of restoring someone to life. It is also a remedy for panic in the doctor, confronted with disaster, now dealing with her own racing pulse and racing thoughts.

UNRESPONSIVE AND NOT BREATHING NORMALLY?
→   Call resuscitation team
→   Start CPR

'Someone get on her chest, for fuck's sake!' Mr Smith was shouting. 'Or do you want me to do it?' I felt the air move as the first doctors on that day's arrest team arrived. 'What happened?' someone said. Seven seconds had passed and 'assess the patient' was finished. No signs of life, no breathing, no pulse. One of the new team put a bag-valve mask on the patient's face and squeezed in two breaths, and I started chest compressions. The song we'd been taught for timing compressions immediately started up in my head. *Nelly-the-elephant-packed-her-trunk.*

As with most resuscitation attempts, the patient remained dead. After twenty minutes the medical registrar called it in a tactful medical registrar way. 'OK, we're not going to win this. Thank you,' she said. Everyone went back to their days. As I came out from behind the curtain I saw the patient in the next bed was crying. The ward cleaner had her arm round the patient's shoulders. Her mop was propped against the wall. 'Don't worry, lovey, that never happens usually,' the cleaner said. The surgical registrar poked me on the shoulder. 'Come on, chop-chop!' she said.

Ward round had a performance element even in the absence of death. The infectious diseases consultant was like a children's entertainer: crumpled trousers, comedy ties, belongings falling out of his pockets. I expected a squirty flower to appear in his buttonhole. He sat all over the beds, which you were no longer meant to do (infection control). Once he sat on an elderly patient's bed and then lay down, hands behind his head. Their two heads on the same pillow looked comical. He prescribed another patient a nightly glass of whisky ('Drambuie 10mls o/n'). He picked up a book from the patient's bedside table and read the last page in silence while his juniors stood waiting. 'Uh-oh!' he said. He rounded in a white coat that was yellow with old age; the sister made him take it off, for hygiene reasons. Some of the other doctors embraced the then still-newish dress code – 'bare below the elbows' – with enthusiasm. One of the gynaecology consultants liked to start his round at the nurses' station in the middle of the ward. He swept off his jacket and flapped it over the back of the chair. Rolling up his cuffs, he rammed the end of his tie into the gap between his shirt buttons. Then he squirted a cupful of alcohol into his palm and gave himself a splashy scrub with it, forearms as well as hands. 'All clean!' he said. 'Now it's time to GET DIRTY!'

At medical school they had briefed us about 'appropriate dress' before we began our clinical placements. We were given a handout which explained the rules. *Please dress smartly and sensibly, remove facial piercings, no denim*, it said. My friend had a tongue piercing; we discussed whether he needed to take it out. 'It's *inside* my face, not on it,' he explained to the lecturer. On our first full clinical day, the male students came to the medical school wearing shirts and ties. They looked younger than they had in their jeans and sweatshirts. The women wore black trousers or pencil skirts and office shoes. We looked like we'd received a mass summons to appear at a magistrates' court.

Once I'd started work it was hard to know who the other staff were. We used clothing and kit as an aid to identification. No one introduced themselves: I don't know why this was. 'Hi, I'm Smith the medical student,' you would say. 'Hi,' said the other person. You were meant to know who they were already. We wore ID badges, but these hung back to front most of the time. You couldn't ask anyone to turn their badge round as that would be hostile. Indeed, even asking someone their name risked sounding aggressive. Why did you need to know and what were you planning to do with this information?

As a house officer, you needed to carry things – a stethoscope, your bleep, your phone, a pen, money for the canteen, and in these olden days, before smartphones, the *Oxford Handbook*. Everyone had a roll of tape, which we used to stick everything to everything: cotton wool to arms, nasogastric tubes to cheeks, scraps of paper into the notes. Edged with fluff, the tape was a linty rejoinder to every hospital campaign about hygiene. It was usual to thread the roll onto your stethoscope or dangle it next to your ID badge, where it would gather more fuzz from your clothes.

As your life was spent either making a list of jobs or updating the list of jobs, you also needed a surface to write on. Some F1s carried a clipboard. 'Secretaries!' we sneered as we crouched by the patient's bed and used the mattress as a desk. Our accessories meant the house officers were easily identifiable. We could also pick out the pharmacists, who were better dressed than us, and carried less stuff. But as the doctors ascended in seniority they shed kit, and it was harder to be sure who was who. Many of the consultants no longer even carried stethoscopes, instead holding a hand out for a junior's if they needed 'a listen'. A person with no bag was likely a consultant, a person with a room of their own.

Some time into my training, a Yorkshire medical registrar called Kate Granger died of cancer. Before she died, she wrote two books about her experience of being a patient. She also started a national campaign called 'My Name Is' to encourage staff to introduce themselves to patients, after she observed that many of the people treating her never told her who they were. Staff started wearing 'My Name Is . . .' lanyards, which hung face-in next to their hospital ID. Now we occasionally told patients 'My name is Dr Smith', but we still preferred to keep such information from each other. Or we stuck coyly to first names, which was unhelpful at times of reckoning. 'Who told you to bring this patient in here?' asked the consultant, enraged at the annexation of one of her side rooms. 'I think he said his name was Brian?' said the F2.

The uniformed staff were equally hard to identify. One of the wards had a chart to help you tell the professions apart. It looked like a field guide to insects, each thorax a different colour – navy polka dots for the specialist nurses, green tabards for the clinical support workers or CSWs. Worst was theatres, where everyone wore identical clothes and covered their faces. Who was the consultant, who the operating department practitioner? Anaesthetists often wore trainers rather than rubber clogs, but you couldn't always see people's feet. It was better to say nothing than to do anything as gauche as ask.

The most certain I ever felt about anyone's identity was during an afternoon of pretending. The A&E I was working in had set up a simulated emergency for teaching purposes. The consultant ran through the scenario and asked us to take our places. He told us to label ourselves with our names and roles. As we waited for the arrival of the actor playing the trauma victim, the senior registrar peeled off stickers and handed them out. We stuck them to our chests. DR SMITH, SENIOR REGISTRAR, MS SMITH, TRAUMA NURSE, DR SMITH, F2. It seemed transformatively sensible, and I wondered why it never happened elsewhere. A few minutes later the emergency phone rang, and the mock-up was ousted by an actual emergency. The air ambulance was coming in to land in the park opposite. We ran outside and saw the helicopter hovering as we waited at the traffic lights. We ran across the road and through the park gates. The helicopter landed and the medical crew and the A&E team conferred for seconds over the stretcher. A&E took over compressions. The crew were terse. We ran the stretcher back across the road and into resuss. The pretend casualty's details had been rubbed off the whiteboard and the real new arrival's written in their place. The patient, a toddler who had fallen from a window, was dead when she arrived, and could not be brought back to life. The registrar came out and took off his sticker and threw it in the bin. He had blood on his scrub top. 'I'm so sorry,' I said. 'Fucking shit,' he said.

For eight years I worked in different specialties and different hospitals. I belonged to one deanery, or geographical region, for my first two years, and I moved to a different deanery when I started specialist training. Each deanery spanned several counties and contained a few hospitals and multiple GP practices. Your posts for the year could be at any hospital or practice within the area. You rotated post every three or four or occasionally six months. Sometimes the new specialty was in the same hospital, but more often the new job meant a new workplace as well. You could request one location over another; for example, you might prefer a hospital that wasn't a two-hour commute from your flat. But it was ultimately the deanery's choice, and you had to go where they sent you. Long commutes were common. Sometimes people fell asleep on the motorway after night shifts. The juniors talked about tactics for staying awake – driving with all the windows open; playing death metal; having someone phone you on the hands-free and talk you home. One morning one of the F2s came in with two black eyes. She had driven into the central reservation on the M1. 'I woke up on the rumble strip,' she said. 'These are from the airbag. It's like being punched in the face!'

As a junior doctor you finished each post on a Tuesday and started the new post, or 'rotated', on a Wednesday – on a night shift, if you were unlucky. Twice my new job was at a hospital too far for commuting, which meant moving house in the twelve hours between jobs. Everyone knew to label the box that contained your bedding in case you only had time to unpack one before you went into work.

The worst of the rotating was that there was no opportunity to communicate with the doctors who had been doing the job the day before you: there was no overlap. They had all gone to their own new posts, taking their priceless knowledge with them.

It was not done to say that any of this was difficult, although you were allowed to express a limited amount of fear. For example, as someone who'd never treated a child, you could state you were concerned at the prospect of starting paediatrics. The rota would inevitably reward this worry by making your first shift a night shift, so that you could be more alone with the sick children. Any attempt to change this would elicit phrases like 'steep learning curve' and 'learning by doing'. No one confessed to fear that they might be too slow-witted or emotional or tired to manage the job at all.

It took eight years (rather than five) for me to complete my training, because I got married and had children and then did some of my posts part-time. I was an F1 in my second hospital post when I met my husband, R. He was an F2, one grade above me in training terms and fourteen grades above me in confidence terms: he was planning to be a surgeon. I had been at my hospital for four months when he began a rotation there. He appeared in the doorway of our ward one day when I was writing in a patient's notes. He was wearing a trilby and a bright pink shirt. The F1s stared at him. 'Pink Shirt Friday,' he said. 'You don't have that here?' We did not. 'Is this where the ward round starts?' he asked. How can he not know the basic information, I thought. Soon my future husband was reprimanded by Sister for writing notes in brown ink instead of black. He was baffled. 'It's Café des Iles!' he said, showing her a bottle of fountain-pen ink. 'It's NHS policy,' she said. 'Get a biro.'

A few weeks later he came to the ward with a coffee from Starbucks. 'This is for you,' he said. I couldn't drink it there: staff were not allowed to drink on the wards. I took all rules extremely seriously. We swiped our way back through three doors to the doctors' office. 'I think you're allowed to *carry* a drink,' he said as I shielded the cup from view. I started going out with him soon after that, although I did not allow him to tell anyone we were seeing each other.

Every evening I went to handover. One evening, as usual, the medical registrar ran through the patients that had been admitted that day. The room was packed with staff: the day doctors, the night doctors, the senior nurses and the bed manager. 'Seventy-seven-year-old male NSTEMI ... Eighty-two-year-old female ARF, CAP ... Sixty-one-year-old male suspected PE,' said the day reg, who was talking very fast. He knew the night reg was unimpressed by the volume of patients we were handing over. As he reached the news that there were also seven patients still waiting to be seen, I heard R calling through the closed door for someone to open it. 'Hands full,' he explained. He was carrying a travel bag. The zip bulged open, revealing a multipack of crisps and the aerial of a portable stereo. 'Nights: got to be ready,' he told the room.

Some things were the same in every post. At the start of every shift I took a piece of paper from the printer, folded it in half and began a job list, each task given its own tick box:

- Mr Smith – Chase bloods □ and CXR □
- Mr Smith2 – Request CT abdo □
- Mrs Smith – Spk family □ ABG □ Spk GP re meds □

Thirteen hours later, at the end of the shift, I fed the crumpled, ticked paper into the shredder. It sometimes had bloodstains on it, which looked fake. I was good at getting blood out of people but still used the even-then-outdated method of a needle and syringe, rather than the 'closed system' where you slip the blood bottle straight onto a cuff on the needle. I filled the blood bottles by puncturing the bottle's vacuum with the needle and letting it suck the blood from the syringe. A drop occasionally dribbled out and reminded me that nothing disperses like blood.

I remembered my first day as a medical student in A&E. A nurse thrust a syringe full of arterial blood at me and told me to take it to the blood gas analyser. The urgency with which she said 'Run!' felt right. Arriving at the machine I discovered that the blood needed to be transferred into a slender glass capillary tube before it could be introduced to the sampling nozzle. Samples must be tested immediately, before they clot. I couldn't work out how to get the blood from the syringe into the tube. I tried injecting it in; blood dribbled everywhere except through the tiny orifice. Panicking, I pulled the syringe's plunger out altogether. This broke the seal and instantly emptied all fifty millilitres of arterial blood over me. Now it looked like a thousand millilitres. It spread and clung like no substance I'd ever encountered. Backtracking to confess, my shoes left bloody footprints across the floor. 'Jesus *Christ*,' said the registrar.

After bad shifts I took my piece of paper home with me, wanting to re-check the check boxes in peace, to see what I had missed. Occasionally I brought other things home by mistake – most often, the bleep. Home after a night shift, I put my hand in my pocket and found three tubes of cold blood that I'd forgotten to put in the chute, the temperamental transport system that carried samples to the lab. It was only ten minutes' drive back to this hospital, but now it was light, which meant visitors arriving and the start of the day shift, everyone showered, undishevelled. There wouldn't be any parking. I got in the car feeling even more downwardly mobile than usual.

It was hard to get through the jobs list without interruptions. If you were handed the crash bleep at the start of a shift, you were part of the crash team. The departing doctor would unclip it and pass it to you at handover. 'It hasn't gone off today,' they would say, or: 'Three arrests – it's been a nightmare.' Sometimes the crash bleep came with a swipe card that overrode the lift or opened every door in the hospital, to allow you speedy access to all areas. I soon formed a specific phobia of being handed this bleep on any new job. This was to do with navigational fears. I started in a several-thousand-bedded hospital on a two-mile-wide site at 9 p.m. The crash bleep went off an hour later, and the verbal message told me to go to ward 11B. I ran, up stairs, down lifts, along corridors. I crossed an empty car park. A rabbit was loping around under the street light. I found ward 11A and ward 12. A porter came to jog alongside me. When I arrived, a clinical support worker was drawing a sheet over the patient's face.

Initially it had troubled me that I often didn't know the other members of the crash team. Now it no longer mattered; I knew they were other on-call doctors. We'd all had the same training. Anywhere you were, the drill was always the same, the steps of the algorithm. Arriving at the bed there was usually a group of staff there already. You could work out roughly who was who from where they were standing (anaesthetics went to the head of the bed as they were responsible for the patient's airway). This time, a thin man stood at the foot of the bed in a blue scrub top and chinos: the medical registrar. The uniform-on-top, regular-clothing-below combination was popular with the med regs, who spent so many hours at work that they metamorphosed into hybrid hospital crea-tures: half human, half beast of medical burden. 'Let's get a gas,' he suggested in the calm way also characteristic of med regs, who generally avoid shouting and panic (or they would spend much of their lives in shouting and panic).*

'I'll do it,' I said, wanting a job. I didn't like watching arrests – if you were on the crash team you had to attend, but sometimes so many people turned up there was nothing for you to do but stand about trying to look relevant. I crouched next to the bed and took the patient's hand. I hadn't looked at her until now. It was a woman, perhaps in her fifties although so unwell it was hard to tell her age, her race, or her sex for sure – I guessed that from the

---

* The med regs attend all the emergencies, and are responsible for everything when the consultant is not there – in the night, half the hospital, including A&E and theatres, will be bleeping the med reg, as will the GPs from the out-of-hours clinics, wanting to send a patient in or some advice about how to keep them out.

length of her dark hair. The woman's face had a blue tinge, and her lips were blue. 'Do we know what happened here?' said the med reg. The healthcare assistant, who had put out the crash call when her patient had collapsed, was crying, touching the corners of her eyes with her little fingers. 'She was fine, she was *fine*, we were talking about *Strictly*.'

As I rotated through the different specialties, acquiring experience and then losing it again, the rounds seemed to get larger and longer. On a liver job we had thirty or more patients to see every day before we could do anything else. 'Come on, come on, come on!' the consultant said as we assembled. The computer couldn't boot up fast enough; the juniors couldn't write fast enough. At each bedside you could feel him twitching.

Most of the patients on his ward were alcoholics. Many were now encephalopathic – their scarred livers no longer able to filter toxins, which instead drifted back to their brains, lowering their consciousness levels like a stroke occurring in increments. Their slurred equivocations had a stereotyped quality, as if they were reading from a script. They shared a habit of exaggerated courtesy: of all the patients I've ever met, these were the only people who really did address doctors as 'Doctor' and nurses as 'Nurse'. Their characteristic response to any question was a silence. After a few minutes they would look into your face. 'What was the question again, Doctor?' They were not the ideal forever patients for an impatient man.

That week our oldest patient was sixty-five. He had alcoholic liver disease, which had caused cirrhosis. Cirrhosis does not usually cause any symptoms until you 'decompensate': that is, your liver starts to fail. The consultant had warned him that his condition would eventually make him ill, but Mr Smith hadn't understood how quickly this would happen. He had felt fine. Until the previous Friday, when he looked at his hand and saw it was yellow. He looked in the mirror and his face was yellow too. He went to Tesco to buy a bottle of vodka. After drinking that he went to A&E. He was the most jaundiced patient I had ever seen. If he held out his hands in front of him, compliantly demonstrating for the medical students, they wagged up and down spontaneously, a sign called 'liver flap'. He was dying. It was too late for a liver transplant: he couldn't go on the list anyway, as he was still drinking. The round stopped in front of him; a circle of doctors, pink, black and brown skin, none of us jaundiced. 'You are making the nails for your own coffin,' said the consultant, tapping his foot.

Mr Smith looked at the floor, and then up at the round. He inspected each of us. 'I am, yes, Doctor,' he said. He died that night.

The next day we arrived at his bed to find a new patient, a man in his sixties who had suddenly turned yellow. 'Decompensated alcoholic liver disease,' said the house officer, introducing the new Mr Smith. He read out the patient's liver blood test results. 'All good, Doctor?' said the new Mr Smith.

The liver ward was near the vascular ward, which was filled with patients who were 'missing bits', to use the registrar's description. I knew this ward well: as medical students we had been sent there frequently to practise clerking. Vascular patients often needed multiple admissions and so were at home in the hospital and made for relaxed interviewees, ideal for students. This was how I met Mr Smith. After many admissions he knew all the staff. He filled us in. 'Mr Smith the vascular surgeon has a short-man complex,' said Mr Smith. 'But at least he moves slowly. Better than Dr Smith Liver: watching him makes me dizzy.'

Mr Smith had had a different body part cut off on each admission. 'Started with my left great toe,' he said. 'It went black.

Looked like a prune.' The vascular ward was situated at the top of a tower block. It wasn't ideal for anyone missing a limb, as most of the vascular patients were. Smith would park his wheelchair next to the lift and wait. With one arm and no legs, he could navigate the lift but struggled with the heavy door at the bottom. With a single hand he also found it difficult to light a cigarette once he'd got outside. So he would wait for passing staff to see if he could cajole someone into escorting him down in the lift and then lighting one up for him. In his prime, before his amputations, Smith had smoked eighty cigarettes a day. 'Barely a break between,' he said wistfully. 'Just solid.'

Vascular disease and liver disease seemed old-fashioned illnesses, from a time when it was normal for graphically terrible things to happen to people – coughing up blood, losing body parts. I thought of the emphysema and chronic bronchitis patients, now labelled COPD, laid out in rows in the respiratory wards. At four in the morning they were all awake, upright in their beds, holding on to the rails, gasping at thirty or forty breaths a minute. The patients tended to be older and poorer, and they had often contributed to their own suffering, by drinking alcohol, or smoking, or becoming very overweight. 'It is not our place to judge,' said the staff, in acknowledgement of all the judgement. Perhaps worst off of all were the patients with non-alcoholic liver disease or non-smoking arterial disease: tarnished by association, like non-smokers with lung cancer. These illnesses didn't seem to have charitable campaigns or cute logos (what would they use, an amputated foot? A blackened lung?). 'Nobody cares, darling,' an old man with COPD told me. His lips were mauve from low oxygen. 'It's just old fellows coughing and dying.'

As a student, I had liked vascular disease, as the pathophysiology was straightforward and the outcomes described in pictures.

Arteries that were slowly furring up gave you pains in your legs when you walked – 'window-shopper's disease'. An artery that was blocked suddenly gave you the '5 Ps': a limb that was pale, pulseless, paraesthesic, painful and perishingly cold. As a junior doctor I never saw the vascular surgeons or their patients any more. They were tucked away in their surgical subspecialty, while I rotated through medical jobs, the busy unsorted catch-alls: acute medicine, care of the elderly, general paeds. Until one night something went wrong with one of the patients' legs on the medical admissions ward.

Earlier that evening one of the house officers had asked for help. He had failed to get a blood sample, so he had called me, next up the chain, his senior. Mrs Smith's veins were tiny. She was angry at having been pricked so many times. She showed me her bruises, which were dramatic black weals, as elderly people's often are. She didn't want any more attempts. I told her that we thought she might be in kidney failure and that we needed a sample to see how her kidneys were. We agreed I would have one go only, and that I would try her femoral vein, which is a big vein deep in the groin. It is surprisingly less painful than poking about in wrists or elbows.

I palpated for the pulse of the femoral artery. Nerve-Artery-Vein-Y-front I said in my head, to remind myself of the location of the femoral vein in relation to the artery – medial, not lateral. I got twenty millilitres of dark venous blood on the first strike. The patient felt nothing. We shared relief. I took the sample to the doctors' room to package up the bottles. Half an hour later, the patient started screaming, a noise you rarely hear on the wards. 'My leg! My leg!' she was crying. I ran back to her bed and pulled off the sheet. Her left leg was white. It looked as though someone had put an artificial limb in the bed with her. I ran back to the office and bleeped the vascular registrar. He came in minutes, saw the patient for a minute, and minutes after that the patient had been wheeled out by porters who were running, which you never saw. She was going for emergency surgery. I was sure I had destroyed her leg.

The registrar frowned and whistled when I told him what had happened. 'Bad ... very bad,' he said. He started to write in the notes. I watched his bent head. And then it was the only time I ever cried in hospital – two tears, which fell out although I tried to suck them back into my eyes. They stung on my face. I had sixteen patients waiting to be seen. 'Oh, my dear, I am *teasing* you!' he said when he looked up from the notes. 'It is nothing to do with your blood sample. It is just bad luck. I am pulling your leg. Luckily you still have one.'

There was no escaping phlebotomy, or cannulation, or NG tubes, or catheters, but I disliked doing more invasive procedures. Too much infringement on other people's bodies. 'I can't do that, sorry,' I told an obstetric consultant who had suggested I do a caesarean section; she was convinced (as surgeons often are) that anyone can do these simple operations if they concentrate. I probably did have the technical knowledge to do a section by then, as I had assisted in twenty or more while working as an obstetrics and gynaecology F2. But I didn't want to. The magnitude of the surgeon's role in someone else's body still shocked me, and my imagination tortured me with potential complications. In my timidity, I was unlike any doctor that I'd ever read about. Mikhail Bulgakov sawed off a farm girl's leg when an emergency amputation was required, although he was only twenty-four and filled with the knowledge of his inexperience, the only doctor for miles, in a landscape containing wolves. At thirty-four, in a hospital near the M1, I couldn't see myself performing an emergency amputation.

I didn't much like sticking things in or taking things out. In hospital, procedures were viewed as the fun part of the job,

offered to the juniors as a treat. 'Mr Smith needs an ascitic tap –
fancy that?' said the registrar, radiating generosity. I went to see
Mr Smith, to explain what I was planning to do. I always let
these conversations go on too long, as I tried to postpone the
moment of doing. When I reached Mr Smith's ward the nurses
said he was 'away with the fairies'. He was lying in his pyjama
bottoms, skeletal except for his abdomen, which was swollen
with the abnormal collection of fluid called ascites. He looked
like a drawing of a fat stick man. I showed him my trolley of
equipment and explained the plan. We needed to get a sample
of the ascites to see whether it had any cancer cells in it or cells
suggesting infection. 'How lovely, darling,' he said. 'Do you want
me to hold anything?' I went back to the registrar and explained
I'd only done one ascitic tap before, and did he want to come and
supervise me? 'See one, do one, teach one,' said the registrar, a
phrase you hear a billion times a week in hospital. 'You should be
on "do one", if you've done one already.' I agreed that I should.
I continued to stand near him in silent hope. He ignored me. I
went to the patient's bed and started tipping the equipment onto
the sterile trolley. When I looked up again the registrar was
standing there with his arms folded.

The patient began a story about a man he had known who
looked like the registrar – 'Same little beard, but he was taller
than you ... broader as well ... more muscly?' This friend, the
patient said, had ended up friendless and alone. 'Even his dog
didn't want to be with him any more.' The registrar ignored both
of us. I swabbed the skin of Mr Smith's distended abdomen and
prepared to stick the needle in. To do the procedure, you have to
go straight through the wall of the belly at a right angle to the
skin; it looks dangerous. You shouldn't hit any organs because in
the ballooned-out abdomen they get pushed to the back by the

pressure of the ascitic fluid, and your needle is poking in through the front. 'Just remember not to kebab anything,' said the registrar.

I rotated on. The respiratory F2s rushed to put in the chest drains, and the surgical F2s jockeyed to go to theatre. I did the ward rounds and sorted out the discharges and clerked in the new patients and put in the cannulas and helped the F1s with the blood-taking and updated the drug charts and checked the blood results. I started new medications and stopped others. I responded to emergency bleeps and routine bleeps and bleeps where the person on the other end denied having bleeped. I learnt about what people look like when they're ill, and what people worry about when they're sick. And I learnt about contemporary medicine's favourite topic: communication.

Talking to Patients

My medical school taught an integrated course where we were exposed to patients (or they were exposed to us) from the first term. This was unlike traditional medical degrees, where you did a few years of theory before being allowed into a GP practice or a hospital. The idea of the integrated course was that you would combine theory and practice from the start, rather than spending three years on the science of medicine before discovering on your first hospital placement that you didn't like patients. As integrated students we spent one day each week on a module called clinical skills, which was taught through lectures, seminars and role plays. The role plays were pretend consultations in which you learnt the correct words and behaviour to encourage your patient to divulge more information ('go on' was a recommended phrase; 'OK, OK!' wasn't). Every lecturer opened by asking you to guess how long most patients talk before the doctor interrupts them. They all had different answers, but it approximated to about seven seconds. We were meant to be aiming for something called 'the golden minute'; the theory was that if you could remain silent for this long, the actor-patient would crack and pour out the tale of spousal disharmony and trouble at work that was underlying his complaint of 'headache'. Whenever I inflicted the golden minute on real patients, they looked disconcerted. At this point in my training, no one told us that some doctors got only ten minutes in total with the patient, and that you would therefore be unlikely to spend a tenth of it on silence.

We made videos of ourselves consulting, which were shown to the class. Things we liked to do included: swinging on the back legs of the chair; clicking the top of a pen; twiddling our hair; staring at everything in the room other than the patient's face, or conversely staring so intently into the patient's face that you could see her edging her chair backwards or fiddling with her bag in an effort to break eye contact. We cleared our throats. We scratched. We yawned. We sighed. We said 'OK?' at the end of every sentence. After some training, we gathered we were not only meant to be empathic, but that we were meant to *demonstrate* empathy. To do this we inserted the phrase 'that must be very hard for you' into any available pause, even if all the patient had said was that 'it's itchy'. We also prefaced every question with a question. 'Do you mind if I ask you a question?' we said.

We were also meant to learn how to close an interview without being brusque or dismissive, and what to do if the patient grew angry and started screaming 'You're all the fucking same! You're a fucking waste of space! This place is a fucking joke! What the fuck is the point?' as a man did during one of my placements. The F1 told the angry man, 'I can see it must be very hard for you,' to which the patient responded, 'NO YOU FUCKING CAN'T!' before stalking off down the hospital corridor muttering 'sanctimonious arsehole'.

On placements we practised our interview skills on patients. It was always described as 'a chat'. 'Why don't you go and have a chat with Mrs Smith?' the registrar would say. Off I'd shuffle to Mrs

Smith's bed. I'd clear the box of tissues and the bottle of squash off the chair next to her pillow and sit down. Then I'd introduce myself: 'I am a medical student' (it was only years later that I realised that many people have no idea what this is – are you training to be a nurse? A university lecturer? Have you already qualified?). I turned my notebook to a clean page and wrote MRS S and the date. I drew the symbol for female and wrote 'DOB' followed by Mrs Smith's date of birth, as I didn't know any medical acronyms yet apart from RTA (road traffic accident), SOB (short of breath) and MI (myocardial infarct). Mrs Smith had kidney failure, so I wouldn't be needing any of those. 'So, when you got your diagnosis – I understand it must have been very hard for you – how did you feel?'

It was an interesting system for learning, as the patients said what they liked. They couldn't be coached, and we couldn't be supervised – there were no spare doctors to supervise us. During my psychiatry rotation, interviews were predictably unpredictable. It took forty minutes by bus to reach the psychiatric hospital. The windows fogged a few minutes after leaving town, so that the hills outside disappeared. Inside the hospital, all of the outside disappeared – there was a shortage of windows looking out, although all the doors had one for looking in. I tried not to think about the metaphors. My first interview was with a fifty-year-old woman with bipolar disorder, who was currently manic. I waited in a room for the nurse to bring her in. 'You think you're the fucking queen of England don't you,' she said as she sat down. 'Nice little middle-class girl with her little notebook. All ready to do your best for Teacher. Ah, Queenie, you don't need to blush! Am I making you uncomfortable?'

Common themes emerged. Power was being manipulated. Information was coming in. Poisonings were occurring. The hallmark of psychiatry interviews was the extremely rational nature of some of what the patients said. We had been taught that moods could be contagious – that you might feel high after encountering someone high, or low after interviewing a patient with depression. But you could also have your factual convictions picked at until you felt uncertain. Penetrating divinations were mixed in with delusions, and many of the patients, living as they were in an upregulation of emotion and a downregulation of rules, were skilled readers of feelings. Specifically, they were expert detectors – and creators – of embarrassment. 'You loved yourself a little bit when you put that shirt on today, didn't you,' a patient said to the consultant. 'But did anyone else love it? Does anyone else love you?'

You couldn't always know if what the patient was saying was true or not. A delusion is a belief that is not shared. There was a lot of scope in this definition. It was easy at this point in my training: we were in a psychiatric hospital with locks, alarms and surveillance windows; you could make assumptions. Later I had to diagnose people on my own, without a massive prompt from my surroundings. At a GP practice, a man came to see me every week for months. He was upset about his next-door neighbours. They were playing loud music and having loud arguments. 'They're driving me mad,' he said. Then a housing officer phoned, wanting to speak to a doctor about the patient. There was information she needed to pass on. I explained I couldn't give her any in return; she sounded irritated, as everyone always does, but decided to share her news anyway. The patient had been phoning the council repeatedly about the noise, she said. She had gone out to investigate. 'The next-door flat is unoccupied,' she said. 'There's been no one there for six months. I went there myself at night, and listened for an hour. I also put a thread on the door so I could see if anyone had broken it.'

'Do you usually do that?' I asked. 'Put threads on doors?'

'He is very convincing,' she said. 'I thought I was going mad.'

The medical school curriculum put neurology into the same rotation as psychiatry in a way that made only anatomical sense. We visited a residential home for people with spinal injuries. Spinal injuries are often young, healthy people's disasters, acquired in the course of fun, of joy or adventure – riding a horse, diving into a swimming pool, climbing a rock face, trampolining. In a moment fast is turned into slow, active into sedentary, fit into unfit. Many patients shared the same final memory of flying through the air. Now you became a patient with a number and a letter, labelled with the level at which you've damaged your spinal cord. This delineates your degree of paralysis and hence the definition of your life's new abilities, what you can or cannot do: L1, able to use a toilet independently; C8, able to use a fork; C3, needing a ventilator.

Before we went to speak to the patients, we had a tutorial. They are not patients, they are *clients*, the nurse told us, unrolling a long poster of a spine. He whacked the spine with the edge of a ruler to show us possible bisections and counted down the vertebrae from the top. 'C1. Quadriplegia. Can't breathe unaided. Superman's injury.'* We were in the occupational therapy room, surrounded by the clients' art. There were enchanted kingdoms with turquoise waterfalls and emerald forests done in bright acrylics. The paintings rested against the walls and in a stack beneath a long horizontal window, which was filled with a view of the sea. No one had painted the view. 'They don't like real,' said the nurse.

I went to speak to one of the clients. Her room was tiny. She sat in her wheelchair and I sat on her only chair. There was a bed, a

---

* Christopher Reeve fractured C1 and C2 – his top two vertebrae – in a fall from a horse, and was afterwards quadriplegic and breathed via a ventilator.

hoist, a TV and a sink. 'I tried to kill myself as soon as I'd got off the ward. As soon as I'd got this room,' she said. 'Tried to drown myself in the sink. Fucking impossible. I ran the tap and when it was full I put my head in the water. But then I didn't have the neck strength to keep my head under.' I sensed she wasn't meant to be telling me this. It was like when they invited a palliative care patient to speak at a seminar, to dispel our prejudices about dying. When someone asked him what dying was like he said, 'It's shit.' No doubt medicine had created categories for this: depression of terminal illness; mood disorders of the spinally injured.

We weren't always on our own: sometimes we went to clinics, at the GP or the hospital, to see how doctors talked to patients. There was rarely enough space in the consulting rooms. We wedged in next to the waste bin or sat on the examination couch, dangling our legs while trying not to dangle them too actively. One afternoon a consultant told us that wriggling in her clinic was bad form. It reminded her of 'too much face-acting' among the extras at the opera. 'I don't want to hear any rhubarb-rhubarb either,' she said.

'I've never been to the opera,' the other student said in my ear.

'No rhubarb-rhubarb!' said the consultant.

Sometimes the doctors forgot we were there. I went to sit in Dr Smith's gastroenterology clinic. He arrived five minutes later, carrying a foot-high stack of notes with a cheese bap balanced on top. His first patient of the afternoon was already lingering outside the door, anxious that I'd taken her place. Dr Smith reassured her. 'I've got a student with me today, do you mind?' He began his consultation. 'So, take me back to the beginning. Right ... right ... and you've had that for how long? Right ... right ...' Once the patient had left, Dr Smith pressed his Dictaphone up against his mouth and started to dictate. 'This young woman came to see me complaining of *blah* stop she has some family history of *blah* comma and *blah* stop I have arranged for investigation into *blah* and she should come and see me again for results stop yours sincerely.' He turned and skimmed the notes through the air, aiming for a pile behind me. They glanced off my head. 'Sorry! Didn't see you there.'

Starting work in the hospital laid waste to our communication techniques. No one cared what you did with your pen, your hair or your empathy, and no minute was golden. One evening, writing drug charts at the nurses' station, I looked up to find a patient waiting in front of me. She was wearing a cashmere sweater over her pyjamas. 'Gin and tonic, please,' she said, placing a hospital beaker on the counter. We both looked at it for a moment. 'I'm afraid we're out,' I said. 'Can I fetch you some water? Tea?' 'Tea,' she said. 'Do you have any Earl Grey?'

The next day I took some students to interview Mrs Smith about her stroke. She was washing her hands when we arrived. She turned the tap off and shook her hands over the sink. Then she walked up to one of the students, tugged his shirt out of his trousers and dried her hands on his shirt tail. 'Now, what can I tell you baby doctors about?' she said. 'She thought I was a towel!' I heard the student saying afterwards.

'Do you mind if I ask what kind of accommodation you are living in?' I asked patients when I was at medical school. In A&E this became a checklist. 'House or flat? On your own? Stairs?' The patients had their own scripts. Nights in the hospital could acquire a carnival air, as the patients with dementia woke up. Like everything in medicine, this had a name: sundowning syndrome. Dusk agitated the Alzheimer's patients, even if they were living in the electric light of the hospital wards. In their homes, nightfall caused increased confusion. 'Mr Smith, seventy-year-old male.

Found in the street trying to saw through a lamp post with a butter knife,' said the paramedic, handing over. I went to clerk Mr Smith. He was skeletal, his pyjama trousers pleated and secured with a safety pin. He didn't seem confused.

'Have you been losing weight?' I asked him. He said he hadn't.

'What did you eat yesterday?'

'Something from the Co-op,' he said. 'It came in a box, that you put in the microwave, so I put it in the microwave. Heated it up. Well. It wasn't at all what I was expecting. I was expecting roast lamb, peas, sort of a taste. Gravy. I can tell you, it wasn't like that at all.'

'So what's brought you in here?' I said, switching to the kind of open question that was meant to yield informational gold (although by now I already knew there was a group of patients who would answer this with 'the bus!', 'an ambulance!' or 'you did!').

'Oh no. That is a complicated business,' Mr Smith said. 'Have you checked under the cushions?'

It was particularly difficult to tell people bad news. A suggested format for how to do this (and how not to do it) is taught in most British medical schools. It is a topic: breaking bad news. The rules were common sense. You had to find somewhere private and quiet, give a colleague your bleep, turn off your phone. You needed to try to discover how much the person you were talking to knew already, to avoid giving a biopsy result to someone who didn't know they'd had a biopsy. Then, the warning shot: 'I'm afraid I have bad news.' A pause for the implication to sink in. Then the facts; although, just before the facts, you needed to check with the patient how much they wanted to hear, as you weren't meant to press death on people who didn't want to know about death. You were to avoid delivering a mass of information to someone too upset to take anything in;

using vague, misleading or medical language; offering misplaced reassurance. In role plays at medical school this was easy, as you informed a fellow student that you were sorry to say they had cancer. In reality, it was fraught.

I found that the temptation to avoid bad words was strong. I might start gently, mentioning a 'shadow', a 'patch', or a 'funny spot' on a scan, with the intention of later converting these words into less ambiguous ones. If the relatives said 'growth' I said 'growth' too. But then you got stuck – a warm feeling would develop between you as no one mentioned cancer. It was difficult to break this. But the too-thorough application of checklists felt glib: bad newsiness. The undertow of insincerity could not be cancelled by overuse of the 'oncologist's head-tilt', or by patting the patient an excessive amount.

Hospital life made things difficult. Most of the time you had to speak to people on the ward, or sometimes in the corridor, as it was quieter.

At four o'clock one morning I watched a man die. The clinical support worker had bleeped for a doctor before she realised that the patient had a DNAR – a Do Not Attempt Resuscitation order. The patient had asked us to fill it out. He had brought up 'The Form' as soon as he'd learnt his cancer was incurable. 'This is good learning,' said the registrar as we went to his bed. I'd stood twisting my legs round each other while she explained the form to him. It wouldn't affect his treatment in any way, we would still try to mend any problems just as we would for any other patient. But if he were to die, 'If your heart were to stop for any reason,' said the reg, we wouldn't carry out chest compressions or administer an electric shock or adrenaline. Mr Smith thought this sounded fine. He was tired of being ill, he said; when death came, he wanted it to happen without interruption.

He had been an inpatient for a month. He had had an operation that had not worked, and had been nil by mouth ever since, fed by a tube into his stomach. I saw him every day on ward round, where I mainly wrote 'obs stable, P: continue' in his notes. I visited him many times in between, to take his blood or replace his cannula or arrange his investigations. At each visit he told me what meal it was about to be, or what meal had just passed, and we imagined what food he would have eaten. He wasn't a fancy eater even of fantasy foods; he mainly ate imaginary meat, potatoes and toast. Once he sat with his eyes closed while I put in a new cannula. The crook of his elbow was white with scars. 'What are you thinking about?' I asked.

'A boiled egg,' he said. 'I didn't even rate them that much. Now I'm thinking: perfection.' His hands were so thin that the tendons stood out like an anatomy drawing. Back when he'd been well, he told me, he'd been a great cyclist. One dawn when I had been called to his bed (his breathing always got worse as the sun came up) he told me that he'd once cycled through the night to visit his son, who lived on the east coast. He'd got there just as the sun was rising over the sea.

In the past week he had developed pneumonia. None of the treatments we tried made any difference, and soon he asked us to stop checking his bloods and then he refused his antibiotics. His organs started to fail, and when the CSW came to do the night observations on her other patients, she saw he was unconscious. She put an oxygen mask on his face and went to bleep the on-call F1, which was me.

When I got to his bed, I saw he was dying. There was no way to alter this. I took hold of one of his hands and the CSW took the other. We looked like we were having a prayer meeting. Mr Smith's breath came in deep, irregular gasps. His lips were changing colour despite oxygen. 'Shall we take the mask off, Mr Smith?' I said. I lifted it off, trying not to drag the elastic on his hair. He had always hated it when we gave him oxygen. The nurses had phoned his family, but they had not yet arrived. The pauses between his breaths got longer and each time I thought, This is it, but it wasn't, until at last there was only a pause that extended until it was clear that he wasn't going to breathe any more. I put his hand back on his chest and gave it a pat.

I went out of the ward and took the lift down into the lobby, which was empty as it was so early. I thought I would go outside for a minute, walk a loop around the outside of the hospital and then go back in to do some of my jobs before I verified the death. Through the glass door I saw two women by the intercom and then I heard the night security guard behind me. As he went to let them in, I saw it was Mr Smith's wife and daughter. I thought of turning and running up the stairs, like when you see someone you don't want to see and suddenly become absorbed in striding to your destination. It is easy to pretend urgency as a doctor in hospital; people imagine your life consists of urgencies, so they expect to see you running or looking distracted, fulfilling your role. I went over to the women and saw that they recognised me. This was not the place to tell people bad news, in an empty hospital vestibule with one of the lifts occasionally landing and sliding its doors back with a ping as it did all night, even when there was no one in it.

'What's happened? Please can you tell us what has happened?' said Mr Smith's daughter. Her mother was holding the big flower-print tote she brought in every day. I imagined it sitting by their front door at home, ready to go to the hospital again. How was I to delay the news until we had got in the lift, gone up to the fourth floor, turned into the corridor, walked to the end of that, opened the doors to the ward and found Mr Smith's bed? I could not chat to them about nothing for all of that way. 'I think we should sit down,' I said. 'I don't want to sit down, as that will mean he is dead,' said Mrs Smith.

A few weeks later I had to tell a family about a death that we had not expected. The patient had been admitted earlier that day feeling unwell, although his numbers weren't bad; he wasn't feverish, or short of oxygen, but he looked ill. We admitted him to a ward while we arranged a chest X-ray and waited for his blood results to come back. His daughter went home to fetch his belongings. Without ever complaining of pain or saying anything much at all, his heart stopped. The crash team tried to resuscitate him for thirty-five minutes but failed. We didn't understand ourselves what had happened to him – a silent heart attack? A pulmonary embolism? His family arrived before the consultant had reached the ward. The registrar was at another arrest. The family wanted to see their father right away: I couldn't see how to stall them. I took them into a side room and asked a nurse to come with me. She offered them a drink: a cup of tea? orange squash? The nurse's hands were shaking. No one wanted any-thing. We all sat down. I thought I was going to be sick. I had to check who everyone was – you're his son, you're his daughters, is that right? 'What have you understood about what has happened so far today?' I asked. 'We know he's ill, but he's not that ill,' said a daughter. 'He's really well usually. Are you telling us he's worse?' 'I'm very sorry to tell you that I have bad news,' I said. I forced myself to wait, to let this register. I tried to look into three people's eyes at once. 'He's worse? He's gone to intensive care? You are not telling us he is dead?' said the son. 'I am so sorry, I am afraid he is,' I said. It sounded ridiculous, pure carelessness on our part, as though we'd mislaid him. 'But I don't understand.

What the fuck happened?' the son said. He was crying and the daughters were crying. The nurse sat next to me and I could feel my shoulder shaking against hers. 'I'm so sorry, but I'm afraid we don't know what happened,' I said.

Leaving Hospital

When the time came to pick a specialty, at the end of my F2 year, I chose an unspecialty. I decided to apply for general practice. Although most of my training had been inside a hospital, I wanted to go outside again. I couldn't choose one organ or one system to specialise in. A colleague had opted for respiratory medicine. 'At last I'm going to know something *properly*!' he said. He was excited. I could see this was the path out of ignorance and doubt – imagine how much you would finally *know* about the lungs – but how much would you also miss out on? When I contemplated each specialty I could only see omission – no babies, no children, no men, no elderly.

I liked that GPs were meant to know their patients; it seemed humane, the way medicine should be practised. I liked the importance they placed on clinical skills, on history and examination, which they appeared to prioritise over investigations or tests (at this point I hadn't understood that investigations and tests were not available as freely as they were in hospital). I liked the idea of coming off the rota, of never saying the word rota again. I had spent all the training Christmases in hospital, and although I enjoyed the porters wearing elf ears, I felt I was going to be allocated the Christmas shift for ever.

I didn't know much else about the job, not as much as I knew about all the things I'd learnt that I would now no longer need to know. It was hard telling the hospital doctors when they asked. They seemed to find general practice unsavoury. Although we had been coached to stop being so obvious in our prejudices, the common understanding of GPs as failed consultants lingered. Like all hospital stereotypes, there was truth in it. People did switch to general practice after realising that there was never going to be a post in their over-subscribed specialty or after failing their exams. Or they thought it was more compatible with family life. The few GPs I met didn't seem to find it particularly compatible with family life, but I chose not to hear this. In hospital we had on-call shifts called 'long days', which lasted twelve or thirteen hours. These were recognised as tiring, and after a batch of them you were allocated a day off to recover before going back to 'normal days'. 'All the days are long days,' a GP told me. 'There are no normal days.' I felt she was probably just inefficient. Their patients were mostly well; what could take up so much time?

In hospital we never saw any GPs. We didn't know what they did, or how they worked. Sometimes their patients arrived in what we regarded as an 'unsorted' state and immediately generated lots of jobs – X-rays, ECGs, blood gases. 'GP is an idiot,' said the registrar, hanging up after an outside call. 'Hasn't even done baseline bloods.' Why didn't the GP get some blood there and then? That's what we would have done. I was constantly taking blood in hospital. I bagged up the samples and put them in the collection bucket on the nurses' desk, which the porters emptied several times a day. Or we posted them into the chute. The results were available in as little as an hour later, if the chute hadn't jammed. We didn't understand how things worked outside. We didn't know that GP appointments are too short for phlebotomy, so the patient must make a separate appointment to have their blood taken by the healthcare assistant or the practice nurse or the phlebotomy clinic. There would be no point in taking blood on the spot anyway, as most practices' samples are collected only once a day, by a van that tours the city picking up from each surgery before dropping everything off at the lab. I had never noticed the vans before, although once I knew what they were I started seeing them all the time, and each time I saw one I thought of all the little plastic bags full of blood and urine and faeces knocking about inside.

When the patient arrived, I looked at the letter he'd brought from the GP. 'Dear colleague,' it said. 'Thank you for seeing this seventy-six-year-old gentleman who presents with ...' I scanned the page for the information we needed: the patient's usual medicines, his ongoing medical problems. The letter was printed, which meant it was legible but unreliable. After the GP has typed some text, software autopopulates the remaining fields. The resulting problem list can look a little random:

- Underwent a Test
- Superficial Laceration
- Wished to Discuss Sterilisation
- Tired All The Time

'All I want to know is if this heart failure is new or not,' said the registrar, holding his hand out for the letter. 'Echo Performed,' it said; the system had not imported the result.

But we could not complain, as sometimes the patient came with a handwritten letter and nothing else. If they had been admitted in the course of a home visit, the GP could not access a computer, although again I did not realise this. I thought some GPs simply did not like typing.

> Dear Colleagues
> 76 yo male – ?acute heart failure.
> O/e RR28, bibasal creps.
> Thanks & bw

The paper was dimpled from where the GP had used the side of her bag as a desk to lean on. Sometimes it carried a smell of the patient's house: cigarette smoke, dog, washing powder.

At the end of his stay we discharged the patient back into the community with a letter. The letter was not always synchronised with the patient; once the human had left, their paperwork lacked urgency. All the discharge letters included a section labelled something like ACTION FOR GP, in which we listed some jobs for the GP to do. 'Please arrange an OGD/an X-ray/check the bloods/titrate the medication', we typed. It didn't occur to us to explain why any of these things needed doing – perhaps we thought the GPs would know intuitively. The community seemed highly random to us. One morning, the F2 told us about his recent post in general practice. A patient had produced a bundle wrapped in tissue and asked him to take a look at it; the F2 had been reluctant. 'It's usually shit,' he told us. But it was a ping-pong ball. 'I think it's a pigeon egg. It needs to go somewhere warm, if it's going to hatch,' the patient had said. 'Can you put it somewhere warm?'

My understanding of general practice was mostly derived from childhood. I forgot that a GP had recognised my brother was ill and admitted him to hospital: the hospital was more memorable than anything that happened before it. But I did remember going to the doctor myself, usually for tonsillitis, which I had several times a year. Mum took me one day after school. The waiting room smelled of TCP. Everyone was coughing. I coveted the magazines. The GP wore glasses, which seemed right for a doctor, and she frowned as my mother explained the history. It wasn't clear if she was disapproving of us or of the illness for having the temerity to recur. She stuck a tongue depressor in my mouth when I was just starting an 'ah', making it clear that she was in charge. Another time I had a rash that Mum thought might be measles. The GP took a book off her shelf and paged through it, looking for some matching skin. There were some nasty rashes in the world. After having a look, the GP wasn't sure what the rash was, but she was sure it wasn't measles. We tried to avoid such uncertainty in hospital.

To become a GP I had to get a place on the GP vocational training scheme, the GPVTS (it has since been renamed GPSTS or GP specialty training scheme, in an effort to boost recruitment). Once you had a place you became a VTS doctor, or a GP registrar. The scheme consisted of three more years of jobs in hospital and in GP practices, which together would add up to being trained. I sat an admission exam and then attended an interview round. Once on the scheme I continued to go to work, and most of the work was still in hospital. I rotated through jobs as before, except now I belonged to the cohort of GP registrars and it was clear to the hospital trainees that we had different goals, and that one of those goals was to leave.

We had more teaching than the hospital trainees, perhaps to compensate for the hours of work we were doing that were now irrelevant to our future jobs (every blood sample, every cannula). For teaching we were released from our various posts to an office block outside the hospital. It was nothing like the GP surgeries or the hospital. There were no stains on the carpet tiles, the windows gleamed and the computers worked. At morning break there were urns of tea and coffee, and snack packets of biscuits, confirming the specialist trainees' suspicion that we had access to superior refreshments.

Each week we worked through the GP curriculum, which can be summarised as 'everything that can go wrong with the human body and mind'. Sometimes we had PowerPoint presentations, often given by ourselves; sometimes we were sent to work in small groups. These were called 'break-out groups' – we loved jargon almost as much as we loved acronyms. In our break-out groups we were meant to discuss the medical topic of the day – incontinence, for example – rather than share stories of how we were being overworked and underloved in our practices or at the hospital. 'I get that ENT is useful for GP, but *this* ENT is *not*,' said one of the trainees about her hospital post. 'Like, when am I ever going to do a Rapid Rhino in the community?' (A Rapid Rhino is a brand of cotton tampon that you stick up a patient's nose to abort a nosebleed. In my own ENT job I did several a week. I have never done one since.) We acted out consultations ('break-out group role play'), with one person being a patient and another the doctor and a third person taking notes ('I liked how you brought up his erectile dysfunction'). We did quizzes, for which the prize was a bag of sweets. It was like medical school except more ambitious. One week we would have a seminar about breastfeeding; the next it was diseases of the ear.

On starting my first post at a GP practice, everything was new again. It was impossible to relate it to hospital. The patients had taken off their gowns and their pyjamas and got out of bed. This was in itself enough to make us suspicious – surely all of these people were Medically Fit for Discharge?

We divested ourselves of our bleeps, our scrubs and our rolls of tape. Now you could put on a watch and a ring and unroll your sleeves; you could wear any kind of shoes as you were unlikely to drop a needle on your foot and no longer had to run anywhere. I remembered one of the F1's on-call socks. 'Look at that cushioning!' he'd said, taking his foot out of his shoe to show us his reinforced heels. You could walk miles on call. Now our on calls were sedentary, and you could wear anything. Nail varnish, Birkenstocks, clogs, a cocktail dress. A GP came to give us a lecture in a knitted waistcoat and hiking shorts.

You will need to learn this computer program, said the manager at my first practice. Neither of the two programs used in English general practice resemble anything devised by Apple. The GP assigned to be my trainer opened his screen to show me the software. 'This is *not* intuitive!' he said. He sounded impressed. Every piece of information ever entered by any healthcare professional unrolled in an endless scroll. Except for anything that had taken place in a hospital, as the hospitals kept separate electronic records. Tiny icons lined all four edges of the screen. I wondered what the designer's brief had been: perhaps someone had requested a visual interpretation of generalness. It was difficult to find any particular piece of information, and sometimes there were mistakes. The data is only as good as the person entering it, said everyone.

Sitting in a room was novel. It was disconcerting to be stationary after years of movement. Consultations felt different without an audience. In hospital, with its thin curtains and crowds of staff, everyone knew what you were doing, and although the old 'firm' structure had been fragmented by the change in working-time law and new shift patterns, you still belonged to a team. Now I sometimes had observed surgeries, with my trainer watching me, and I sometimes hosted a medical student in my room, but most of the time I was on my own.

It was true that the days were long days, between ten and twelve hours. I arrived at half-past seven to start the paperwork. The first patient was booked in at eight-thirty, the last at ten to six. At this practice there were sixteen face-to-face appointments in the morning and ten in the afternoon. At the end of each clinic there were phone appointments and home visits.

There was a lot of correspondence. As juniors in the hospital, we had never received letters. Occasionally you were allocated a share of a pigeonhole, in which you occasionally found a pharmaceutical flyer. In GP, the correspondence stacked up. Every day the administrative staff scanned in new letters and sent them to your inbox. A count appeared at the bottom of the screen, ticking up through the day. A number next to this tallied the incoming blood results; another counted your internal messages, or 'tasks'; another your pending home visits. If you opened and dealt with the letters, actioned and filed the blood results, went on and wrote up the visits, and carried out the tasks you could shrink each number to zero, but not for long. More paper correspondence landed in your own dedicated tray in reception. The doctors turned these trays upside down before they went on holiday. I thought of Lucy's kiosk in the Peanuts cartoons: The Doctor is OUT.

Letters came from everywhere. From patients, the hospital, the podiatrist, the optician, the schools, the health visitor, the physiotherapists, the community mental health team, the chiropractor, the DVLA, the DWP, social services, the coroner. 'Please can you prescribe . . .' 'Please can you monitor . . .' 'Please can you advise . . .' Is this patient fit to work? To drive? To fly? To do an ultramarathon? To do an A level? Can you tell us about their health issues going back to 1982?

I tried to 'be assertive with the admin', as my trainer suggested. I read the hospital letters as soon as I got to work and carried out lots of ACTIONS FOR GP. Next, I worked through the bloods, cherry-picking those that I could file as NORMAL NO ACTION NEEDED. But often you needed to know the rationale for the test in order to make sense of the result, and this was difficult if it had been requested by a colleague who was now off duty. Mr Smith's haemoglobin was now 80 grams a litre (normal would be above 130 g/L). How urgent was this problem? Had Mr Smith's blood count slid down slowly and predictably due to chronic illness, or was this a new finding indicating he was bleeding to death on his bathroom floor?

I kept forgetting the prescriptions. The electronic ones created their own score, but it was on a different part of the screen that failed to catch my eye. We still got paper scripts too, green bundles that needed checking and signing. 'A taste of fame,' said one of the GP partners, autographing a stack at lunchtime between spoonfuls of Pot Noodle. But you couldn't scribble if there was a query – now you needed to scroll through the notes again to find out why this Mr Smith was on so much diazepam or whether his aspirin should have been stopped.

Throughout the day the nurses and the healthcare assistants put their heads round the door, or sent messages that popped up on the screen. Can I have a signature? There is someone on the phone who ... Do you think this leg is infected? Could you have a look at this ear? Reception rang. The paramedics are on the phone. A pharmacist is on the phone. A consultant is on the phone. The police are on the phone. About six times a week, some common drug went out of stock and the script came back with a note requesting an alternative. I prescribed an alternative. The script came back again – not in stock, please prescribe another alternative.

I had started reading *A Fortunate Man*, John Berger's classic account of the life of John Eskell (called John Sassall in the book), a GP who worked in a rural practice in the Forest of Dean in the 1960s. The book is illustrated with photographs taken by Jean Mohr. In Mohr's photographs, Sassall is never smiling. His brow is very creased. The book pays little attention to Sassall's wife or children; no domestic woolliness is allowed to sully the intensity. He entered general practice as a single-handed practitioner, with a list of about two thousand patients. Having previously been a naval surgeon, he prefers action:

> He had no patience with anything except emergencies or serious illness ... He dealt only with crises in which he was the central character: or, to put it another way, in which the patient was *simplified* by the degree of his physical dependence on the doctor.

As time goes on, Sassall changes. He doesn't encounter patients as incidents any more, but as people with stories, who alter through time. The patients start to talk to him and tell him things. 'They, as they became more used to him, sometimes made confessions for which there was no medical reference so far as he had learnt.'

This felt familiar. There was no medical reference for a lot of what we saw, and we found this disconcerting. In hospital you could keep things doctorly: arrange a blood test, organise a scan, consult another specialist. But community patients were a different population, where you could not assume that everyone was ill.

General practice was assertively clinical. From medical school onwards we had been told that ninety per cent of the diagnosis was in the history. If you'd asked the right questions and listened to the responses you should arrive at the answer. The examination and any investigations were just to confirm what you already knew. In hospital we had not always respected this method. Doing a test was often quicker than teasing apart what a patient meant by 'it's sort of in my chest, but also sort of in my throat'. But in GP we had to go back to history and examination, as it took time to arrange investigations and longer to get results. What exactly was the patient trying to tell you? What could you see and feel and hear? You had to make a working diagnosis quickly, as there was nowhere to store the patient while you pondered. But you also had to understand the limits of a single appointment. Sometimes it was OK to be inconclusive. A viral illness, a sprain, a harmless rash: all would get better with time. The patient was to come back if it did not. We learnt this as a strategy called 'time as a tool'. It was often resented by patients, who preferred speedier and more tangible tools.

In hospital the patients were largely pre-sorted. They had something wrong with a system or organ and they belonged to a specialty. Even the muddle of A&E patients had self-identified as having a problem that was urgent, or they came with clues – a strong smell of alcohol, a finger in a plastic bag. But no one organised GP patients into handy groups like this: that was your job. Everyone came to the GP. Some people were ill, but many were not. Often people came because there was nowhere else to go: there was not much available for patients with mental health problems until their mental health problems got bad enough for inpatient treatment. There was even less remedy for what we called 'social issues': loneliness, poverty, bad jobs, bad housing. 'SLS,' my trainer said about every other patient. He meant Shit Life Syndrome. 'Very hard to treat.'

I felt more in demand than I had in hospital, and less in control. 'See your GP,' said every newspaper article and every charity campaign and every phone advice line. We had complicated the situation ourselves by encouraging patients to attend for problems that were not yet causing problems. We wanted to diagnose and treat high blood pressure and cholesterol and pre-diabetes before they caused any symptoms. In Sassall's time, people didn't go to the doctor to preserve their future health. Now we raised awareness and ran campaigns to try to prevent illness before it occurred.

The contrast between Sassall's doctor's life and my own ran abrasively through my thoughts. I coveted his knowledge of procedures. He attends every birth in his rural community, and most of his patients' deaths; the photographs show equipment, interventions. It was a time and a place where the GP did minor surgery and obstetrics as a matter of course. The first thing Sassall thinks when he hears of an accident is that he has left his stretcher at the hospital. I tried to imagine owning a stretcher.

Sassall did both more and less than contemporary GPs. He would have had only a handful of drugs for illnesses such as diabetes or depression or rheumatoid arthritis. There were fewer diagnoses and fewer treatments. Heart patients were heart patients: they did not have one of two categories of heart failure, a choice of coronary stents, three or more types of pacemaker, a range of anticoagulants. None of Sassall's patients would have been on twenty-six drugs simultaneously. Many contemporary diagnoses – fibromyalgia, CFS-ME, POTs, ADHD – did not exist in a formal sense.

Sassall had no patients like Mr Smith, my fifty-year-old patient who had a cancer that the oncologists called 'treatable but not curable'. Smith had been terminally ill for months. The chemotherapy had caused painful ulcers on his toes. 'Fingerless socks,' he explained, when I came to his house on a visit. He had seen me looking at his feet; I was trying to understand how his heels were dressed but his toes were bare. He had cut his socks in half. At night he put his feet in a cardboard box and draped the duvet over the top. He showed me the boxes that had failed their auditions – too tall, too wide. I admired the arrangement. 'Going to need a bigger one soon,' he said. I laughed before I realised what he meant and then had to try to take the laugh back. We had started a syringe driver – a portable intravenous medication pump – for him, as his nausea meant he could not manage tablets. While the medication dripped into his arm, he worked on taking tiny mouthfuls of build-up drinks, his only calories. He got thinner and thinner and all he complained of was feeling cold. He sat so close to his electric fire that his legs developed the lacy rash called erythema ab igne: a historical kind of affliction. He outlived any prognosis he would have received in Sassall's time.

I envied Sassall's confidence. He suffered from anguish throughout his life, but his role at least was clear. The community knew who he was and what he could do for them. Perhaps there was more acceptance of limits. When I tried to explain limits, specifically the limits of medicine, it was an unpopular topic. Everyone expected to get better: unwellness was unacceptable. 'Something has to be done!' the patients said. Many people didn't like doctors, which meant they didn't like me. I was a representative of things that upset people: professionals, the state, mainstream medicine. 'Do you not know *anything* about nutritional yeast?' said a patient. 'That is not the correct way to assess the thyroid. You're checking the wrong parameters,' said another, passing me a printout. 'Doctors never understand how to do this properly.'

At my first practice, I looked after Mr Smith, who was disabled by arthritis. He lived by himself in a studio flat. He no longer slept in his bed, as getting out of it was too painful, instead spending his nights in a chair with a duvet over him, homeless in his own home. One wall of his sitting room was taken up by a mirrored wardrobe which had a crack running across it where he had fallen on it. He had taped the crack with strips of masking tape to stop the glass from falling out.

He was not pleased to see me. The new pain medicine wasn't helping. No, he didn't want to change it to anything else. No, his mood wasn't good; how would my mood be if my only excursion was a weekly trip to Lidl on a mobility scooter? 'He doesn't like doctors,' one of the partners said when I got back to the surgery. I saw Mr Smith every few weeks when he called for a visit. Each encounter followed the same format. He would open his front door and immediately turn and hobble into his sitting room. There we would sit reflected in the mirror, the jagged crack running between us in an obvious manner, while he went through a tally of that fortnight's disappointments. His back, his hips, his heartburn. None of them improving, which proved that medicine was useless. He saved me pages from the tabloids to prove how suspect medicine was. He explained general practice to me. All we did was stare at computers, he said. We couldn't do proper medicine or we'd be hospital doctors, SPECIALISTS. We were obstructing his access to X-rays and MRI scans. Furthermore, they had employed too many women, which meant there was now a problem with staffing due to everyone being part-time. 'True, true,' I said.

'He never separates an illness from the total personality of the patient – in this sense he is the opposite of a specialist,' says Berger of Sassall. I knew I was the opposite of a specialist, but I still wasn't sure what that was. 'GPs are experts in people,' a lecturer had told us one day. It seemed a bold claim. I was beginning to discern trends in people, if such a thing is possible, but whenever I thought I'd identified a category and placed a patient into it, the patient showed me I was wrong. I thought of all the elderly people I was meeting, many of them widowed. Widowhood was not a subject I'd encountered much before. Now it came up often – women live longer than men.

On my first week as a registrar, observing a surgery, an elderly patient came in wearing a matching hat, shoes and earrings.

'Our number-one patient, aren't you, Mrs Smith,' the GP said.

'I'm ninety, you know,' she said.

'You're not really ninety.' He looked at her notes on the screen. 'You are! Bloody hell!'

She had brought a sheet of paper with her blood pressure readings written on it. She also wished to report her indigestion. 'I had whitebait yesterday for lunch and it was still repeating on me at bedtime.' Dr Smith reminded her to take her Gaviscon. My boy used to take that, she said. And his dad. Suddenly they were talking about her son, who had died from cancer in his fifties. 'He was the same age as my father when he went,' said Mrs Smith. 'They die, the men, but we go on and on.'

Soon I had widowed patients of my own. Mrs Smith was eighty-five. Her husband had recently died of lung cancer. He had never acknowledged his illness, continuing to walk to the newsagent every day even when his lung function was down to ten per cent. Finally he became too breathless to leave the house. He had read the same newspaper for forty years: the newsagent started a round to deliver just his paper. I had only met Mr Smith a few times, but I remembered him leaning out of his chair like a child in a buggy, tethered by his oxygen. Mrs Smith came to the GP every week now for 'check-ups'. I think she was partly proving her ability to leave the house, and partly testing whether contact with the doctor would harm her, if it would lead to some diagnosis and then further sub-diagnoses, I'm afraid it is cancer, I'm afraid your lung function has deteriorated, I'm afraid you need oxygen, I'm afraid we're running out of options, as we'd said to her husband. 'I never went anywhere near a doctor for years, and now look at me,' he'd said when I visited. 'Can barely pull my own trousers up.'

'I can't decide whether he's sailing a dinghy or flying a plane or climbing a mountain now,' she said, a few weeks after his death. 'I know he's not sitting on a cloud, at any rate. He hated sitting.' I know he did, I replied. He liked to be on the go. She looked at me. 'You're a good doctor. When you look at me I can see you are looking right into my soul.'

The other Mrs Smith had brought her husband for an appointment every fortnight. He had been unwell for almost ten years. Whenever I spoke to him, he would look at her, and she would repeat what I'd said in exactly the same words but with her own choice of emphasis. At last he died, and I didn't see her any more. A few months later the practice asked her to make an appointment to discuss her blood test results, as her cholesterol was rising. 'Your cholesterol is quite high,' I said. 'If we start some medicine now we might be able to lower it, which can be helpful in the long run.' She put her hand on mine. 'May I swear, please?' Feel free, I said. 'I don't give a flying fuck.' Fair enough, I said.

'Now he's on the other side of the door, I can't see the point of being here. Without Dad.' Dad was her husband. 'I can feel him waiting for me on the other side of the door.'

'Which door is that?' I said, ridiculously.

'Any door, darling. I can hear him breathing. You know he was a noisy breather.' She patted my hand. 'That's enough of your time taken.'

We had been trained not to make judgements, to be aware of our own prejudices, but we had also been encouraged to summarise and to categorise. It was hard to work on pattern recognition without forcing everything into patterns. 'Who knows what "gestalt" is?' a lecturer said to us one day. It emerged that the lecturer didn't know quite what it was either. 'It's an unknowable thing,' she said eventually.

I looked for what the trainers called 'soft signs' of how the consultation was going to go. I developed a fear of patients with folders, particularly ringbinders with subject dividers: they did not fit into ten minutes. Once a couple came in and they both had notebooks. They sat down, opened the notebooks, uncapped their pens and looked at me. I didn't know where to begin.

My relationships with patients were often less straightforward than they had been in the hospital. I hadn't realised how much people alter the truth. Now I was frequently having a new kind of communication experience based on knowing I was being lied to but not being able to express this knowledge. Accusing people of lying was rude and hostile and liable to bring you a complaint. Most of the untruths were with the intention of getting hold of drugs to use or to sell. We would consult over the lost prescription, which was only ever for benzodiazepines or opiates – no one lost their blood pressure tablets. I tried to enjoy the creativity. Lost it at my sister's; lost it on the bus; fell in the river.

'You dropped your prescription in the *river*?'

'It came out of my pocket as I cycled over the bridge. I was like, oh shit, not again, they're never going to believe this.'

A bottle of morphine 'fell off the top of the washing machine during the spin cycle' and smashed on the floor. The bottle was always full when this happened. Sick notes, now renamed by the government but no one else as fit notes, were another source of woe. One day I took my children to the swings and saw my patient, crutches discarded, diving after a football. I stood behind the slide and contemplated the next consultation without enthusiasm. I realised there were a lot of professions where people lied to your face – the police, lawyers, traffic wardens. Even teachers assisted their pupils with the trauma of lost homework. It was just how the world worked. It still hurt my do-gooding heart that the patients thought I was stupid.

Some mornings or afternoons I was on call. The on-call GP was responsible for all the day's unforeseen events. You needed to ring back and triage the incoming phone calls, and be available to everyone who needed a doctor – emergency patients, the medical students, the practice nurses, the hospital, the paramedics. On the appointment screen, the afternoon was a tower of pink blocks that were continuing to stack up. So far I had nine patients to see and fourteen phone calls to make. One of the blocks turned purple, which meant it had been booked as a home visit. I hoped no more would turn purple. At this practice, reception printed out the visit requests and put them outside the doctor's room. I opened my door and picked up the sheet. 'Pt not herself', the receptionist had written. The patient was eighty-eight years old. 'Not herself' is a broad complaint with a diagnosis ranging from irritable to dead. I phoned the patient. It went to voicemail. I rang back every half hour through the afternoon, between the other calls and consultations. Reception phoned but couldn't get through either. We tried the patient's son; it went to voicemail. I considered phoning the police, but pictured the patient in her sitting room, too peacefully deaf to answer the phone, and her door being broken down and her house full of uniforms. I finished seeing patients at ten past six and the last phone call at seven. I got in my car and put the satnav on. She lived on a post-war estate, low brick houses set back from the road. Up Primrose Lane, down Willow Road, to Sycamore Drive. I strained to see the house numbers in the dark, then got out of the car to check I had the right house. The front door had a glass panel through which I could see the light was on, which was good: dark houses in the dark are unnerving. I held my phone up as a torch over the key safe and typed in the number on the visit sheet. I opened the door. Hello, Mrs Smith! I called. It's the doctor!

There was a bed against one wall of the sitting room, covered in a green blanket. It was very warm, and the television was on. An elderly Caucasian woman in a bobble hat was lying in the bed. 'Hello!' I said. 'I have no idea who you are,' she said. 'I'm the doctor! Your carer called us; she was worried you weren't feeling well.' 'Oh,' said Mrs Smith. She had round pink cheeks; with the hat and the blanket pulled up to her chin she looked like the wolf in *Little Red Riding Hood*. I started a history, but she couldn't give me a history. 'Do you know where you are?' I said.

'I'm in my house. Do you know where *you* are? You're in my house as well!'

'Where's that accent from?' I said.

'Beijing,' she said. I felt this probably wasn't true.

'Does anything hurt?'

'No.'

'Can I examine you?'

There was a tray table over the bed with three beakers of tea on it, a paper plate full of crisps and biscuits, and a pair of glasses. Three beakers of tea meant carers three times a day. These were my detective skills. Mrs Smith could not sit forward so I listened to her chest from the front. Her arms were folded in tightly and I had to pull her elbow open to make enough space to put the blood pressure cuff on. 'I'm sorry,' I said. On the television a man was threatening another man with a gun. When I pressed on her abdomen she shifted a little. 'Does that hurt?' I said. 'No,' she said. 'I'm wondering if we might need to get you to hospital,' I said. I was always recruiting this we, the army of righteous doctors.

'No.'

I looked at her. She looked at somewhere in front of her. I didn't think she could see the television without wearing her glasses. The man had been shot and was lying on the floor with blood underneath him. He would need a stretcher. Dr Sassall would have had one; he would have known what to do. I went out to my car and phoned the son again. He answered with his mouth full – suppertime. I mentioned Beijing, and the carer's concerns. 'She's fine,' he said. 'That sounds like her normal self, she doesn't sound ill.'

Occasionally I spoke with members of the community care team: the district nurses, the midwives, the specialist nurses, the physiotherapists and the occupational therapists. At some surgeries things are less fragmented, but everywhere I worked the care teams had been detached from the individual practices and re-formed into areas or districts. Sometimes the district nurses ran in to collect a sample bottle or a signature, but never for long enough that I knew who anyone was. I read their entries in the notes, which I admired. I particularly venerated the heart failure nurse, who was incredibly thorough. If I referred a patient to her she would always 'get him sorted', as we'd said in hospital. She would weigh him and examine him and go through all of his medicines and talk through all of his concerns. 'Lovely woman,' Mr Smith said when he next came to see me. 'Likes everything tidy.'

The practices held multidisciplinary team meetings or MDTs to talk about patients who were housebound or dying. We assembled in a non-timely fashion: the doctors late due to surgery over-running, the nurses late due to traffic and parking. As soon as we sat down everyone pulled out their Tupperware and the smell of food filled the room. We discussed what we thought the patients needed and who was going to do what. Once we'd eaten our lunches everyone began to fidget, the nurses needing to continue their rounds, the doctors their surgeries and visits. I tried to convey gratitude although I rarely knew who anyone was. Without them there was no primary care; in fact, there was no care at all.

When I was still in medical school, a district nurse took me out on a visit. It was a rural practice, and we were going out to a retired postman who was now housebound. We drove a mile up an overgrown unsurfaced track; we were in *A Fortunate Man*. The patient's house was surrounded by fruit trees. Now he could no longer pick them, the apples were rotting on the ground, giving off an alcoholic smell. The house looked very dark; it was a tiny cottage with small, deep windows. 'Make sure you look before you sit down,' the DN said to me in the car. 'And don't breathe through your nose.' The postman came to the door and then hopped ahead of us into his sitting room. He turned on the light, which didn't make anything much brighter. He sat on a kitchen chair and put his foot up on a stool. The DN knelt on the floor. She unwrapped his leg and a smell of decomposition filled the room immediately. 'It's terrible, I'm sorry,' said the postman. 'You'd think I'd be used to it, but I can't stand it.' His ulcers were dripping green fluid. I could look at his leg without sensation, but the smell made me retch. I breathed through my mouth. 'Rotting apples, rotting legs,' said the DN, back in the car.

Most illnesses unfolded slowly, but sometimes there was an emergency. They were less common and less expected than they were in hospital, which meant there were fewer people around to help, and no crash team. Dialling 999 brought you an ambulance, but these sometimes took a long time – hours, even, unless the patient was unconscious or dead. 'Is he awake? Is he breathing?' the ambulance operator asked. You had to say no to one or both questions to get something quickly. Once, a patient came into the room and I noticed he looked blue. As I realised something was about to happen, something happened. He collapsed, falling forwards as I went to catch him, hitting his head on the corner of the desk. I had to ignore my instincts – that is, ignore the sudden stream of blood, which was distracting me from starting with A, B – Airway, Breathing – and insisting I jumped ahead to C, Circulation. The disaster was easy as the patient was unconscious, and when reception called 999 the ambulance came quickly and took him away. I put a wad of paper towels over the blood to soak it up. When I put the paper in the bin, there was a new black stain on the carpet.

My colleague picked up a baby to examine her, and the baby stopped breathing. A man had a cardiac arrest in the car park. But the slower disasters were worse, where you failed to realise you'd missed a clue until hours or days afterwards. One of the GPs told me about her case. I soon realised she was telling everyone in the surgery about it, the Ancient Mariner rehearsing his guilt. On a recent winter afternoon she had seen an elderly woman who said her spirits were 'drooping'. The GP documented this in the patient's own words, as we'd been taught. Had she ever felt like hurting herself or killing herself, asked the GP. No, said Mrs Smith, she could never do that to her children. The GP started the patient on an anti-depressant and typed a referral to old age psychiatry. She suggested a lunch club. A fortnight later Mrs Smith came for follow-up. She said she felt a bit better. She hadn't been to the lunch club.

The psychiatry appointment had not arrived when Mrs Smith went to the railway track and lay down on it and was killed by a train. The day before her suicide she had made an appointment to see the GP but hadn't kept it. Reception marked her slot as a DNA (did not attend). We are taught to check our DNAs to make sure there is nothing to worry about. If a child or a vulnerable adult has not come in, you should try to find out what has happened. On this occasion, the GP hadn't remembered who Mrs Smith was and hadn't opened her notes to check. Or she had checked the notes but not registered the significance of the DNA. Or she had checked the notes and forgotten to phone her. A hundred patients later and the GP couldn't remember what she hadn't done. She had been called to attend the coroner's court. We tried to reassure her. 'If you had rung her she might not have picked up,' we said. 'She might not even have wanted to kill herself then, how can you know?' I didn't try to find out, the GP said. I didn't try.

In the absence of catastrophe there were shocks. As a final-year trainee, I had a patient who seemed subdued. He had recently come out of prison, which fact I was trying to keep out of my brain in an attempt at professional neutrality. 'He's served his time,' my brain kept inserting, like a country and western song. I have forgotten why the patient came in – his symptoms got lost in the static. I was doing my best active listening, nodding, leaning forward, asking open questions. He suddenly pulled his chair right up to mine. I felt panic. He yanked open his shirt like Superman. A button flew off and landed on the floor. There was a twenty-centimetre scar across his abdomen. 'I slit my belly from here to here,' he said, pointing at his scar. 'And I'll do it again right here and right NOW if this shit isn't sorted out.' Afterwards it was hard to reconcile the pantomime acting with the reality of the scar. The next patient had itchy ear canals and also thought she might have athlete's foot, and also she had noticed that she always had to wait at this practice, did I know she had waited twenty-six minutes?

As first-year GP registrars we had started out with twenty minutes for each appointment. The practices reduced the times as we became more experienced, to fifteen minutes, then twelve, aiming for the goal of ten. Time was literally closing in. It was all we could talk about at our teaching sessions. One registrar was using an egg timer, and another had set up her screen to show a countdown timer. 'Isn't that like having an unexploded bomb in your room?' someone asked. 'On ten' did not seem attainable or indeed possible.

Once I was finally on ten, I had to try to stay as close to ten as possible. If I didn't, the day fell apart. Most people were too polite to say anything, but they looked uncomfortable, or sighed when they came in. The parents with children were ragged from entertaining in a confined space. The babies were ratty and hard to examine. But I still couldn't see how to fit a new diagnosis of cancer, or a suicidal man, or a bereaved elderly woman into ten minutes. Even minor skin problems took at least twelve, if you wanted to find out why the scabby baby was not getting better or to stop teenagers with acne trying to scrub off their spots.

I had grand intentions when I started *A Fortunate Man*. I hoped to learn from Berger's reflections on doctoring and community. But I was soon sidetracked by the patients' histories. The book opens with a woodcutter having a terrible accident. Sassall rushes to attend him in the foggy wood. He devises a tourniquet, gives an intravenous injection, and gets the man to the hospital. Berger doesn't tell us the outcome: we never learn if the woodcutter loses his leg. I couldn't think of anything else. Nothing abstract seemed relevant beside the recurring problem of each day: what to do now and what will happen next.

I had started to find my personality problematic. Being professionally gentle was making gentleness feel false. Every time someone told me I was a lovely doctor, that I 'really listened' or 'really cared', or reached out to hold my hand, I felt a glow of satisfaction then instant revulsion. Why was I taking pride? Or sucking up relief from other people's suffering?

I wasn't sure if I was really caring, or performing caringness. I would take the patients home in my head and wake up thinking of them first, just as I had done in the hospital, but did this mean I just wanted to get things right, was I more worried about my own role than about their well-being? In the room with a patient, I responded with an empathy that I didn't have to think about. But when I thought about the encounters afterwards, I felt suspicious. Wasn't this just wanting to seem lovable? Wasn't empathy a way of becoming necessary, a source of power?

I would wake up irritable. Every weekday morning was the same. I got in the car and drove for a few minutes until I reached that day's traffic queue, where I spent the next fifteen minutes. For three months I drove with the *Goldberg Variations* playing on the car stereo. Tears flooded hammily into my eyes as soon as I switched it on. Then it was a month of Bach cantatas. I played one repeatedly, listening for a pause in the music that communicated to me more than the words, which I did not understand. Every day the amount of unknown increased, as the patients appeared at fifteen- and then twelve- and then ten-minute intervals with symptoms that might be something or nothing, how could I know for sure, not that I was even meant to aspire to certainty as a GP, but rather balance or control the level of risk. A lot of my consultations at this time consisted of interpreting pauses, as many of the patients did not speak English, and the interpreters were not always reliable. I would listen for the gaps, and watch people's faces, to try to see what was mattering to them. It was a strain for everyone. The need to be understood made people frustrated. Sometimes they cried.

I picked the Bach out by the pictures on the CD boxes; I could not remember the number of the cantata I liked. Numbers had never had much traction for me. It was always a handicap, but now in GP it felt dangerous. In hospital I prescribed a small number of familiar medicines, and there were nurses and pharmacists to check what I'd prescribed and who would bleep me if I got anything wrong. Now there were hundreds of drugs, many with unfamiliar trade names, sometimes with no more description from the patient than 'it's a pink tablet'. Doses varied for children, the elderly, for people with kidney problems or liver disease. To prescribe, you clicked on a drop-down list that offered twenty or more options. As soon as you picked a drug, a dialogue box popped up with a list of interactions and warnings. Some were obscure, some were important: it was not possible to read them all. I used the calculator on my phone to check every dose I was unsure of and sometimes even doses I knew to be correct. But I could not check everything.

It was almost time for my final GP exams. No one could talk about or think about anything else. First there was a written paper called the acquired knowledge test or AKT. Then it was time for the final clinical exam, the clinical skills assessment or CSA. 'The CSA is like an OSCE, only worse,' one of the graduating registrars told us. Like every other British doctor, I had sat OSCEs – objective structured clinical examinations – throughout medical school. They assess your ability to carry out clinical tasks: examining the heart, taking a history, inserting a cannula. In an OSCE, different stations are set up to test each skill and you must complete every one in order to demonstrate your abilities, or inabilities.

OSCEs formed part of my final assessment for my degree. One morning we arrived at the medical school to find it altered. Now every classroom had an instruction card taped to the door, and every room contained an examiner. We were each given a start station and sent to wait outside the relevant room. Eventually the intercom instructed us to START EXAM, and all the doors opened simultaneously and everyone went into their rooms. Each station lasted for ten minutes, punctuated by announcements of FIVE MINUTES PLEASE and ONE MINUTE PLEASE and CHANGE STATION PLEASE. On CHANGE STATION PLEASE all the candidates shot out of their rooms and bolted into different ones.

Some stations contained a real patient, but others were occupied by actors pretending to be patients, on whom we were to demonstrate our history-taking skills. We had learnt during mocks that OSCE actors were sensitive and you needed to be tactful to avoid provoking fury or despair. Some words acted as triggers: it was always better not to say 'complications'.

At other stations plastic medical models were associated with human actors to create chimeras. First, I discussed an actor's earache with him. Then, at a nod from the examiner, I examined the ears of the plastic head set up on a nearby table. 'Is this uncomfortable at all?' I asked the head as I peered into its ear with my otoscope. 'It's fine,' said the actor, who was sitting a metre away. Another room contained an actor with a pair of plastic breasts strapped to her chest. The station required me to uncover and examine these. I palpated the actor's plastic chest while explaining my actions to her. 'That's fine,' she said.

The GP trainers assured us that the CSA was a more refined examination than the OSCEs. All sittings of the CSA were held at the Royal College of General Practitioners' headquarters on Euston Road in London. The fee was just short of £1500. The registrars who had already done the exam were forbidden to discuss the content with us. Instead they shared practical information such as how to find the RCGP building and the location of the nearest Travelodge. I was impressed by a colleague who said he had only been to London once. 'I used to live there!' I boasted. I hoped this might give me some advantage; perhaps my ability to navigate from King's Cross would confer a professional sheen. Everyone said it was a shame they had been so nervous during the exam as the refreshments were great. 'They give you a *selection* of those mesh pyramid teabags,' said one of the returnees.

In the spring of my final training year I applied to sit the CSA. I took the train to London the night before, even though my session was not until the following afternoon. Next morning, I took the Tube to Euston Road. I arrived at the RCGP four hours before the exam. 'You're a bit early,' said the woman on the door. She could not let me in yet. I walked up and down Euston Road. I went into the Wellcome Collection and tried to summon up some scientific or artistic curiosity, but it was all dead. At last it was time, but then we had to wait in quarantine anyway, as the morning exam had over-run. The holding room was packed with trainee GPs, our wheelie bags and our accessories. We had brought water, sweets, Diet Coke, chewing gum, magazines, crib cards, lucky charms, breathing exercises, prayer. Health and scientific rationalism had deserted us. I wondered what number exam in each person's life this was; supposedly final now, although we all must have sat something labelled finals at least once before. The woman sitting next to me went out to the toilet (a minder had to escort her; they waited for you outside the cubicle door). When she came back, she looked pale.

At last we went up to the examination suite. We were not allowed to speak, and I took this to mean we were not to make any facial expressions either, so I tried not to meet anyone's eye. The pale woman was making snuffling noises that sounded like crying. The man beside me had comb marks in his hair and was wearing a silk tie, but then I saw one of the buttons on his shirt was open, and there was stomach visible in the gap. I stared at his shirt to tell him, but he was looking fixedly in front of him. There would be no announcements in this exam, only buzzers: one to tell you to start each station, another to tell you to stop.

Eventually the adrenaline induced an actor's high, and in some of the stations I felt I had never been a better doctor. It was such perfect medical drama, in a series of clean and orderly rooms, purified of administration and typing and, best of all, free from the risk of committing any error that could result in actual harm. One of the actor patients was wearing a beautiful suit, and I wondered if that was part of his character or if the actor liked suits and knew how fine he looked. As we consulted together I felt we were in a play, something fresh and experimental, with the director taking notes in the corner. The actor responded to my cues with touching emotion. At no point did he rip his shirt open.

When they let us back out on to Euston Road it seemed disorganised, with traffic hammering along and people walking in every direction. I looked at all the pedestrians, wondering why they had come and whether I would be able to find out in ten minutes. On the late train home I avoided the table seat, in case I started interviewing the person opposite.

The next day, at work, I was a temporary celebrity. 'She's back!' one of the receptionists said. 'How was it?' It was not fun, I said. 'Not as fun as work!' she said. It took weeks for the results to be published, and I used the time to replay every station in my head, searching for hidden diagnoses. Why had the woman paused before acknowledging she was married – should I have asked more about her husband? When the patient scratched his neck was he in fact hinting at a skin disease? Some of my real patients seemed like bad actors now and I doubted their sincerity. It was no easier to compress people into ten minutes and I thought how much I preferred consulting if you didn't have to type up any notes or write any referrals afterwards.

The results were communicated via our eportfolios, the online journals in which we recorded our assessments and reflected on our learning. On the morning of the announcement you refreshed your eportfolio's front page a hundred times until the section labelled CSA changed to PASS or FAIL. I sat with my laptop on the stairs, not wanting to commit to any room in the house in case I somehow fixed the outcome. PASS appeared on the screen. I refreshed the screen again to check; it still said PASS. I took the computer downstairs and showed it to R. 'Oh, big surprise,' he said.

Passing the exam meant that my training was nearly finished. I understood I was almost qualified now, although I was otherwise the same as I had been the day before. I didn't contain any more knowledge. I treasured my PASS but couldn't understand how something so significant could feel so arbitrary. It reminded me of the sensation I sometimes had at work, dealing out diagnoses as though I was playing Scrabble tiles while the patient waited to find out the score. URTICARIA. ASTHMA. GOUT. COPD. I even got the little flush of pleasure when a tricky one turned out to be right. Even as I had this thought, I knew it to be amoral. How was this different from the surgeon who thought she was God? What arrogance was I masking with folksy board-game metaphors?

Driving to work felt exactly the same. The only change was that I wasn't anticipating an exam any more, but no feeling came in to replace the anticipation. In the run-up to the exam I had swapped music for educational podcasts, intending to revise as I drove. It seemed over-confident to change back now. Today there was a Canadian chiropractor talking about the shoulder. I liked the way this man taught anatomy: he never assumed you knew anything, like doctors did.

The traffic queue was moving so slowly that my engine switched itself off. I could see the driver behind me in the wing mirror – some days I recognised her, a woman who evidently left at a precise number of minutes past the hour, as I did. The drivers were often talking on their phones, though once I saw something I had thought was traffic-jam mythology: a man shaving in his rear-view mirror with an electric shaver. It was nonetheless not much like LA. The chiropractor was still talking. 'I move the arm up and down like a wing,' he said. I had stopped listening. I was idling in a formerly industrial part of the city, not yet reclaimed by cafés or craft beer; concrete from the 1960s, green and orange cladding from the 1990s, a hill on the horizon with its far side invisible to me and likely to remain so. As with every surgery and every hospital I'd worked in, I followed a fixed route dictated by work.

When I worked in Luton, I knew almost every house in one grid of red-brick terraces. I knew where the kitchens were and how to get round the back if the front door wasn't open and where the patient's bedroom would be once I'd got inside. The patient was most often an old person hummocked under a bedspread, paracetamol and a stale glass of water on the bedside table. I knew every bed in two of the hospital wards. And I knew nothing else about the place. I didn't know where people shopped, or where they met for fun, or what the parks were like, or what people did when they were well. I did once go to the covered market and ate the best curry I have ever had from a stand that one of the other doctors, a Trinidadian, had discovered. In my memory the dish was called 'Golden Fish', though this seems unlikely.

Now in a different city, I passed a red-brick Victorian church and then the white mosque from which Bangladeshi taxi-drivers sometimes reversed with God-given confidence into the main road. Then the traffic thinned out and I could drive a little faster, through the area where the Roma Slovak community lived, families walking four or six abreast, taking their children to school. Roma is not a written language, I thought, irrelevantly, every time I saw them. In Eastbourne, the hospital porters told jokes about people from Worthing and I laughed. In Sheffield, the porters told jokes about people from Barnsley and I laughed. What had I become? A racist? I didn't even know where Barnsley was.

Passing my final exam did not ameliorate my daily sensation of ignorance. 'As a GP, you have to know that you can't know everything,' a lecturer had explained during a seminar the week before. My mouth had been full, as usual. How many biscuits had I eaten during my training? 'You have to realise that not every question can be answered,' said the lecturer, not meeting anyone's eye.

I had started to dread my consulting room. It was spacious and well equipped, but it lacked a window. There was a window frame covered by a curtain, but when you drew the curtain there was chipboard behind it (it was an internal window, which looked into the reception). On the other wall was a canvas of a woodland scene. A path through a forest, dappled sunlight, autumn leaves. It had been hung on a nail by the previous registrar, who had perhaps also felt the lack of a window. It was like finding HELP ME scratched into the paintwork with a pin. The irony was so obvious it made things worse. A painted path that led nowhere! A window that wasn't! All emotions seemed synthetic. I had simulated so much empathy there was no real feeling left. One afternoon I had a migraine. It started while the last patient of the day was telling me why she had come in. As she described her symptoms the side of her face was covered in zig-zags. When she'd gone, I was sick in the sink. The next week I went to talk to the practice manager and she moved me to a little attic upstairs. This had a window high on the wall, out of which you could see only the top of a tall conifer, but it was better.

Yet the feeling of being stuck in a windowless room continued: somewhere hot and brightly lit, that came everywhere with me. I was at work for most of the hours of each week, and outside work I couldn't talk about it. The emphasis on confidentiality felt the same as shame; whenever I spoke I worried I was betraying a secret or breaking a rule. Sometimes I spoke to R and I would feel uneasy, as though someone else was listening. When I told R this he said that was no bad thing: at least *someone* was listening.

R was doing a surgical job in another city. We talked on the phone as he drove home down the motorway. He sounded high from lack of sleep. 'Massive haemorrhage,' he told me, describing one of the night's cases. 'Hosing blood.' Why do you always have to say 'hosing'? I said. 'Because it was hosing!' he said. When he got home, he did everything quickly and neatly, as though he was still in theatre. His nails were shining clean. But surgical training wasn't solely about operations: there were forms, and audits, and clinics where the options were limited by algorithms. Operations were not done for the right reasons, he felt, or at the right time; sometimes they were not done at all. Eventually he decided to switch to GP. It was like watching an orange try to turn into an apple. His first GP trainee post was in A&E, and that was fine as he was still surrounded by crises demanding action and sutures. But his first placement at a GP practice put him in a state of confusion that lasted months.

I offered to help. We practised consultation skills using a CSA role play book. 'Try and find out why this matters to me,' I suggested; I was playing Mrs Smith. 'You need to understand my ideas, concerns and expectations.' 'But why?' he said. 'What about *making you better?*' Preventative medicine baffled him: if you were not bleeding out from an aneurysm what need to visit the doctor? One day he rang me from the car park outside his practice. He was discouraged. I have had enough of all this *nuance*, he said.

We took turns to work full-time. On my days off, I looked after the children, who at one and three had their own preoccupations. My daughter liked everything to have a sound effect. My son would get hold of a word and see how far he could stretch it without having to learn any more words. 'Hot!' he said, which covered the sun, the radiator, the bath, food.

I felt solitary and stupid, and now I also felt afraid. It was worst when I was on the different clock of home, which was less pressing and distracting than in the surgery. In the park the children and I looked at the pond, and I quacked at the ducks and agreed it was hot, while my brain considered the options. I was afraid of making a mistake, of injuring someone, of killing someone, of being sued, of doing something wrong and realising it, of doing something wrong and not realising until the letter came through the door from the GMC. I was afraid of ridicule, of judgement, of my ignorance. I was afraid of becoming so tired that I was no longer afraid and so became truly dangerous.

There was a spate of doctors taking their own lives during my training years (the suicide rate among doctors has always been high). I became fascinated with each one, trying to reconstruct their lives, imagining them consulting with their patients, their tenderness, their expressions of concern, while their thoughts recycled the knowledge of the trap they were in. The junior hospital doctors were beautiful and young, and I could imagine how kind and high achieving they were, how shocked by the onslaught of the job, its fundamental undoability. But I was fixated on an older woman, a GP, who had recently gone missing. She had two small children. For a week, she appeared on the local news: a CCTV clip of a woman in a sweatshirt walking down a street. 'Normal, normal, normal,' as my son said when I asked him to describe something. The woman was younger than me, although her youngest child was the same age as mine. Her husband made an appeal on the news; you could see their kitchen behind him, children's beakers in the dish rack, laundry drying on an airer. Not having access to prayer, I was agitated all week, putting the radio on in the car every time I went on a visit, scouring Google when I got home, knowing hope is not medically effective. Eventually they found her body. She had killed herself. There was a campaign to have everyone talk about suicide, around this time, to 'destigmatise' it. Stigma seemed an irrelevance. They interviewed some of her patients on the news. 'She was a lovely doctor,' an elderly man told the interviewer. 'So caring.'

Sassall – John Eskell – killed himself in 1982. I didn't know this fact when I read *A Fortunate Man* – I learnt it through Google afterwards. I took the information badly: even Sassall couldn't make it? 'What is the effect of facing, trying to understand, hoping to overcome the extreme anguish of other persons five or six times a week?' Berger asks. He recognises that Sassall suffers from depression, but can see redemption: 'Sassall is nevertheless a man doing what he wants ... Like an artist or like anybody else who believes that his work justifies his life, Sassall – by our society's miserable standards – is a fortunate man.'

Every working day rammed home my own good fortune: my home, my family, my salary. I wasn't ill, I didn't have to go to the doctor. I had a house and a car, a sofa and a bed. My arms and legs worked perfectly, my children were a good surprise every day. In a house near the practice, I visited an elderly Somali man with cancer. An interpreter came with me. We found the patient asleep on a chair in the kitchen with his head resting on a pillow on the table. When we asked if he would like us to help him to bed, he said it wasn't his turn. He only rented a fifty per cent share in the bed, he said, and as it was daytime his roommate, who worked nights, was currently asleep in it. 'Shameful,' said the interpreter, as we got back in the car.

I don't see what I've got to be unhappy about, I said to R that night. 'You're doing too much thinking,' he said. That is an aggravating thing to say, I said. Things are not that simple. I explained that analytical reflection was an essential part of being a good clinician. I compared surgical training with GP training and described some important differences. 'See what I mean?' he said.

A few weeks later, I visited an elderly man with terminal lung cancer. He was waiting for my visit, sitting on his sofa with a notepad. Next to him he had a folder with all his cancer literature, hospital letters, Macmillan pamphlets with their green bubble writing. A Labrador lay with her head on his feet. His wife sat in an armchair; after five minutes she took away his cup of tea and came back with a new one. The sun shone through the French windows onto the carpet.

I asked about his appetite. He checked his notepad, and I saw that he had been writing down everything that he ate.

'O-eight hundred hours. Breakfast – one egg, toast.'

Was he ex-forces? 'Navy,' he said. 'You don't need to ask about that.' I didn't need to, he was right – I was trying to round out my sense of him before we talked about what I had come to talk about, which was his death. Getting straight on to death always seemed rude.

The visit had been requested by the palliative care nurse, who wanted a GP to speak to the patient about his terminal diagnosis, and make sure all the practical aspects of dying had been taken care of, that the patient had been prescribed any drugs he might need and that the paperwork had been done.

I asked Mr Smith if things were making sense to him so far, in terms of his illness and his treatment; I needed to know how much he knew and how much he'd understood. 'In the booklet, it says that this is a treatment for lung cancer. But I don't have lung cancer any more – Mr Smith cut it out. Now I have liver cancer. So they're treating the wrong thing, aren't they?'

I started to explain cancer, which was ambitious. He passed the notepad to his wife – 'You write it.' I explained mutinous cells breaking off from the main tumour and flying off to different locations via the blood and the lymph, where they then set up new tumours – new camps. Metastases. I knew my personalised military metaphor was lame, and he had the tiniest bit of contempt in his face as he looked at me. 'I think you have several places affected, don't you?' I asked him. His eyes grew wet. 'They can't cure it, you know,' he said. 'It is the end, I do know that.'

The dog had struggled up on elderly hips and was pawing the French windows.

We talked a little more. As I stood up to go, he said something that sounded as though it had come from a book. Patients often use phrases that are familiar from medical dramas – I wondered if we got our scripts from there, if they supplied us with words when otherwise we'd be in a blank cave of shock. No one ever went into hospital, they were always 'rushed in'; and people were forever 'bleeding out'. At the end of the patients' stories of hospital adversity the doctor always said 'you're lucky to be alive'. Maybe we did all say this – all of us alive people are lucky, I guess; all of us, to some extent, fortunate men. Mr Smith took my arm; he wanted me to pay attention.

'I learnt all about the stars and the planets, but I forgot the mysteries within. The human mystery,' he said.

The Mysteries Within

At my medical school we learnt anatomy the traditional way, by dissecting cadavers. One afternoon near the start of the first term, we students went up to the dissection room, the DR. We dumped our bags and coats in the cloakroom and threw away our chewing gum. Then we each took a blue package, which unfolded into a thin plastic apron. The sleeves ended in a hook that went between forefinger and thumb, anchoring them in place – so there's no gap, the anatomy professor explained, between the glove and the gown. No gap, 'because there's quite a lot of fat, and you don't want human fat on your skin, not really. And for that reason also – the fat – it's all right – in the DR but only in the DR – to wash your hands without taking off your gloves. Just give them a little rinse. If things are getting slippy.' A pair of plastic glasses ('you don't want splashes in your eyes') completed the outfit.

The DR was brightly lit, with windows at one end showing countryside with autumn trees. The side windows were opaque glass, to shield the room from view. The doors were alarmed. In front of us were nine metal trolleys with a plastic-wrapped cadaver on top of each one.

The professor was standing next to her cadaver at the front of the room. Behind her was a screen on which the unveiling was to be broadcast. Each group of students had a smaller video monitor above their trolley, showing the same events. Our cadaver was a man aged eighty-three who had died of a heart attack. There was a shallow metal tray next to his swaddled head, containing scissors and scalpels and other metal implements reminiscent of the dentist's, and a small swing bin next to his wrapped feet into which everything associated with his flesh was to go. In a year's time, when our relationship was over, all the pieces would be gathered up and cremated, and there would be a memorial service to which, the professor suggested, we might like to go.

Along the windowsill were jars of old lungs and hearts floating in embalming fluid. The DR was hot, and smelled of formaldehyde and meat, nail salon and butcher's shop. The professor gave us a lecture about behaviour, and respect, and taking care to match body parts to buckets. During this talk she rested both her hands on her cadaver.

'Now,' she said, 'first of all, we're just going to unwrap—' There was a rustle of plastic, and something grey started to appear on her screen. On our table we each took an edge of covering and started to roll it back. There was a crackling noise as the other tables started doing the same thing. We had named our cadaver Mr Smith. His facecloth – a moistened piece of muslin wrapped around his head – was to stay on today. We unwrapped from the neck down. There were more damp muslins under the plastic, to keep the cadaver moist; we picked these off down to his waist. Soon we were confused. The skin was age-spotted and slightly yellow. It really was like marble: cool, with a sheen to it. There was a row of bumps – the ribs – but the torso seemed to be at an odd angle. No one dared say what they were thinking: where are his nipples? For a mad instant I wondered if this was something that happened in death, or old age even. Perhaps it was like Ruskin's shock with the pubic hair, but in reverse – the shocking absence of nipples. Perhaps they atrophy at a certain age, and this is one of those facts that you only learn when you're older. We were too nervous for sense, or to realise that our body was face down.

'Not a problem,' said the demonstrator. 'The surgical guys were doing some stuff round the back, I think. We'll turn him.' A couple of students took a wrapped arm each. I took hold of a leg. It was heavy. It was one thing to be unwrapping a cadaver, and another to be heaving him all over the table. At last the body went over, a hand leading the way; a square of bald, liver-spotted scalp; a large foot with a hairy big toe. At the sunny end of the room a student had fainted.

Our cadaver, like the others, had been brought to the medical school in the back of a chilled van; and like the others, he was valuable. Embalming plus eventual cremation cost around a thousand pounds per body, a bill of about £18,000 for the first year's cadavers alone. By comparison, Donald, the department's life-sized anatomical model, cost £7500 and would last until he broke. But Donald was the glamorous cousin of a shop-window mannequin: perfect, rather than real.

Our instruction card told us to fold back the cadaver's chest wall; that is, to 'deflect the skin laterally'. The skin had already been cut for us, a bloodless line across the base of the neck and a vertical incision from there to the top of the abdomen. We put our fingers in and folded the skin back. The dermal layer was as thick as a paperback. It lay over the cadaver's arm as though he'd put it there himself. Now we could see the pectoral muscles forming two wings over the rib cage. Everything was covered in a pith of translucent connective tissue, through which it was possible to make out some of the skeleton's landmarks. I could see the sternal angle, the ridge in the middle of the sword-shaped breastbone where its two plates, the manubrium (handle) and sternal body (blade) fused together. We put our fingers into the suprasternal notch, the dimple at the base of the neck.

I had the cadaver's cold elbow under my glove. In my head I said sorry. Our group was quickly formulating our own rules. We decided we would not leave our cadaver unfolded, as we'd seen another table doing, walking off to inspect one of the model skeletons and leaving their body flopped open. It seemed disrespectful. Whenever I felt sick, I looked my scalpel and nothing else. You cut things up to cook them, how is this any different, said my brain. A number of differences came immediately to mind. The flesh piled up next to the blade in flakes like tinned tuna.

Years later, I listened to my children discussing a dead bird they had found in the park. 'I saw a dead pigeon today. I saw its meat,' my son told me. R describes the body's contents in the same way. He has retained a sort of butcher's cheeriness, which I think of as the surgical manner. He tells patients that the ache they feel is 'in the meat' of their arm or leg, meaning the muscle or the flesh – as opposed to a malfunctioning bone, joint or organ. He also uses 'unzipping' to mean a laparotomy, the big operation where you cut the abdomen open from the sternum to the pelvis in a vertical line. 'We'll need to unzip you from here to here,' one of the surgical consultants would say, sweeping his finger across the patient's pyjamas.

At medical school they preferred the term 'tissue' to 'meat'. During an anatomy lecture one of the students raised her hand. 'Where *is* the tissue?' she asked. Everyone sniggered, but I didn't know either. In the box of the body, I liked the jewellery – the organs, laid out in my mind like gems on plush, identifiable by shape and colour. Heart, lungs, kidney, brain. Some anatomical structures took a more abstract form for me – anything described as a gland, for example. I could not have attempted to draw one of those. And some were invisible. Could you actually see nerves, or were they sparks of electricity flying about under your skin? To me, an anatomical part was something you could pick up with tweezers during a game of *Operation*. It transpired that tissue could be used as a generic term to refer to any of the body's packing materials – the muscles, the fascia, the fat between organs.

But there were also specific types of tissue. Everything in the body was made of particular kinds of cells organised in a particular kind of way to make up a particular part. So you could have the tissue of the heart, or the tissue of a blood vessel, or the tissue of a nerve. You could see and touch nerves, and even pick them up, I learnt: they ranged in thickness from a strand of cotton to a USB cable.

I found it hard to relate the cadaver to the anatomical drawings we'd been shown. 'Now here's a chap who's had his skin removed!' said the anatomy lecturer, clicking up a slide. It was a delicate watercolour of the contents of the abdomen. At the bottom was the already-familiar signature *F. Netter MD*. Frank Netter trained as a doctor at New York University medical school in the 1920s, but he always preferred art. Eventually, in the late 1930s, he became a medical illustrator for the drug company Ciba. His portrayals of illness embrace drama. My favourite showed a man in a brown overcoat and trilby – an old-fashioned private eye, or perhaps a Cronin GP – emerging from a restaurant into an icy street. One hand clutches at his chest, the other has dropped his briefcase, which is in the process of falling to the pavement. A still-lit cigarette lies on the ground. Snow blows across the frame. In the bottom corner a boxed diagram shows a bare torso with a pink patch shaded across the chest and down one arm, the territory of cardiac pain. I imagined the artist having to snap out of his story to insert the learning point.

As time went on, Netter concentrated on pure anatomical drawing. The first edition of his massive *Atlas of Human Anatomy* (which he called his 'Sistine Chapel') was published in 1989 and it remains one of the best-selling anatomy textbooks. His gouaches, which look like botanical art, were ubiquitous. We all had Netter flashcards: I particularly liked a brain with its territories coloured in primrose, mint and mauve. It was easy to understand what you were looking at when someone had picked out the arteries in red, the veins in blue and the nerves in yellow. But real anatomy lacked Netter's rainbow codes. In the cadavers everything was beige and brown; in CT images everything was black and white. When I saw inside a living body for the first time it didn't look like either.

'What do you think this is?' a surgical registrar asked me. I had gone to theatre to observe an operation. It was the first big surgery I'd been to, and I'd already been surprised by the discovery that intestines are bright pink. I peered into the hole the registrar had made in the patient's abdomen. I could see the liver: brown, with a defined edge like the hull of a boat. I could also see the gall bladder clinging to its underside, a greenish blob like a sea anemone. The surgeon had worked her way deep behind the stomach and was poking at a knobbly piece of tissue with her forceps. 'Think of the pictures you've seen: think, what is related to what?' Looking for a landmark, I finally saw the first part of the gut, the duodenum, which curves in the shape of a C. The unidentified organ had one end buried in this curve, so it had to be the pancreas. In Netter's drawings the pancreas is a plume, like the feather sticking out of a cavalier's hat, its broad end nestled against the duodenum and its long tail pointing towards the spleen. In an actual abdomen, it was a blob: you could see how its name derived from the Greek words meaning 'all flesh'. I had never seen a spleen during dissection – our cadaver's was a shrivelled rag. 'I know it looks like a random piece of meat,' said the registrar.

The surgeons took a practical approach to interior navigation. They often talked about tissue planes, which meant the associations rather than the connections between structures: the 'relationship between the skin of the orange and the fruit inside', as a surgical manual explained. Identifying the planes allowed you to separate organs without damaging them, progress without cutting any-thing, use your fingers to feel where you could pull things apart.

But only the trainee surgeons really needed to know how to cut people up. The rest of us had to be able to locate the body's con-tents from the outside, which was a separate subject called living anatomy. Living anatomy linked the body's interior to its exterior. It identified the surface landmarks of the body and correlated them with the structures underneath. Although I had seen our cadav-er's innards, I still found my own hard to picture. I could feel my breathing, but not the outline of my lungs. I could put my hand on my heart. Of course I knew where my stomach was. (It turned out I didn't. I thought it was behind my umbilicus, the bit you rub to mime hunger. It is actually higher, and off centre, to the left. The kidneys are also about ten centimetres above where people point when they tell you they have kidney pain.)

Living anatomy classes entailed undressing in front of your classmates. Having stripped to swimwear, we were given a set of anatomical notes explaining the whereabouts of different viscera. We had to locate the organs and then map them on each other's torsos with a marker pen. Back home, I found it difficult to scrub the lungs off my back. In general, the sedentary and the women were reluctant to get undressed; we relied on the gym-going boys, who were keen volunteers. Whipping off their T-shirts in a flurry of Lynx, they stood about tautly, encouraging us to shade in their adrenal glands. My understanding of surface anatomy was derived from hairless men with bosomy pectorals (a physique almost never encountered afterwards). Their minimal body fat made finding your way easier, as most landmarks are bony; the prominences and depressions function as a palpable map.

Now when I grew tired of failing to memorise the cranial nerves and rubbed the base of my neck, I felt a bony lump that I'd never thought about before. I now knew it to be the spinous process of the seventh vertebra of the cervical spine. If I found C7 on a patient, I could then count each bump below it and in that way identify every vertebra: Thoracic 1, T2, T3. As the spine articulates with the rib cage, the same method allowed you to identify particular ribs, and the organs beneath. In class, we drew the kidneys, tucked under ribs eleven and twelve. At the front, or *anteriorly*, as I learnt to say, the bony landmarks of the chest could help you find the regions of the heart. I rocked my fingers down another student's breastbone until I found the ridge we'd seen inside the cadaver: the sternal angle. From here I walked my fingers off to the right until they fell into a depression. I was in the gap between the second and third ribs. When I put my stethoscope on this spot I could hear the *dub* of the aortic valve closing.

A few weeks later, the lecturer handed round a set of plastic vertebrae and a Jiffy bag full of rubber spinal discs. A slip of paper stated this was a 'complete vertebral column with sacrum and coccyx'. By now I was seeing body parts everywhere. In the university bookshop they had model ear keyrings for sale, and a pile of cardboard boxes labelled BUDGET HUMAN SKULL WITH REMOVABLE TEETH. Skeletons jumped out at me, posing in chiropractors' windows, revealing themselves with every cartoon lightning strike.

Along with the plastic spinal column, the lecturer had brought a few real human vertebrae and ribs to show us. They were lighter and finer than the plastic models; the groove at the bottom of the rib in which the nerves and blood vessels sit a sharp gutter. When the plastic models grew warm, the real rib remained cool. The original *Gray's Anatomy* describes the rib as an 'elastic arch of bone'. Every bone had its own map; every concavity and convexity had a name.

The anatomy teachers were called 'demonstrators'. They were mostly junior surgeons, teaching for extra income and the opportunity to refine their own anatomical knowledge. After we'd finished our classes, the orthopaedic trainees dissected shoulders and the vascular trainees picked at the blood vessels. The demonstrators appeared to be memorising information as they went. Once I had known that the thigh bone connected to the hip bone. Now I discovered that *the iliofemoral ligament arises from the anterior inferior iliac spine and then bifurcates before inserting into the intertrochanteric line of the femur.* There were hundreds of statements like this. Every muscle had an origin, from a named part of one bone, and an insertion, into a named part of another: the attachments. It sounded like the title of a literary novel. I thought the surgeons were memory prodigies. We had regular memory tests, or vivas, for which we stood in a circle round our body while the demonstrator gave each student the name of a muscle and asked for its origin and insertion. Some of the students stared into the body and others closed their eyes and tried to visualise their flashcards, sometimes resting their hands on the cadaver as if the information might come in that way.

Our lectures focused on parts of particular anatomical interest. We learnt about the eight little bones that make up the wrist (or what anatomy calls the wrist – the widest part of your hand rather than the area under your watch). As with all tricky medical information, the wrist bones had generated mnemonics. Some Lovers Try Positions That They Can't Handle was not the worst. Scaphoid, lunate, triquetrum, pisiform, trapezoid, trapezium, capitate, hamate. The lecturer wanted us to pay attention to the scaphoid in particular, the cashew-shaped bone next to the thumb, which functions like a ball bearing helping the wrist to rotate and flex.

Even this little bone had a relationship to the surface, its own map. We learnt that it lived under a dimple called the anatomical snuffbox. You could find the snuffbox by making a thumbs-up sign and looking for the hollow formed between the two tendons that operate the thumb. In Georgian times people balanced snuff here before snorting it. The scaphoid, we learnt, could be fractured without the patient realising, an injury usually caused by a fall onto an outstretched hand, inevitably called a FOOSH. 'Scaphoid fractures can be elusive,' said the lecturer, showing us an X-ray of the carpal bones. It looked like a bag of marshmallows passed through an airport security camera.

On clinical days we went to the orthopaedic department at the hospital. I felt hopeful: bony anatomy was hard, but fractures seemed more comprehensible, if you ignored the scaphoid. We all knew what a fracture was: usually preceded by an accident, often accompanied by a sound effect. ('You could hear it in the kitchen!' a patient with a broken leg told us. '*Crack!* Like a gunshot!') Outside the hospital, on the pavement by the bus stop, I found an opened cast and a ribbon of bandage lying in swirls. I pictured the patient sawing his way out of it and escaping on the bus.

In the plaster room I watched one of the technicians use an oscillating saw to take a cast off a patient's leg. 'You need to take short, sharp bites, avoiding bony protuberances,' he explained.

He traced a route along the man's leg, naming the bones as he approached them.

We went to see an orthopaedic surgeon operate on a fractured ankle. As she touched the skin with her scalpel a red line appeared, then gaped into a wound a moment later. The surgeon told us she loved this tiny pause between applying the knife and the skin popping open. 'It's like opening a present.' Inside the wound, the tibia was just visible, wrapped in its sheath of connective tissue. The surgeon scraped at the bone to clean it. The fracture, a thin line on the X-ray, appeared as a dark-red furrow through the bone, partly obscured by a scab. Despite anatomy lectures, despite dissection, I realised I still thought of bones as the dry, white items carried round by dogs. In lectures they had told us about bone marrow, how it was not just featureless stuffing but rather a fermenting pool of immature blood cells. The operation made this real. If a fracture tears into the marrow, the bone will bleed.

Later I was sent to sit in the orthopaedic clinic. A man in his forties came in. He held out one shaky arm to be examined and the consultant asked him which tendons he'd cut. I don't know, said the man.

'Can you move these two fingers?' asked the consultant, demonstrating with his own hand. His nails were a manicured pink from scrubbing for theatre.

'Only if I do this,' said the patient, pressing on his palm with his other hand as if operating a button.

'What did you do?' asked the consultant.

'I cut my own wrist. Basically,' said the patient.

The next patient was a teenage girl with her arm folded in a home-made sling.

'How did you do that?' asked the surgeon.

'I punched someone,' she said.

'Right.'

The girl was as matter of fact as the doctor; they could have been two surgeons consulting together. After she'd gone, the nurse said she was unusual, that this wasn't ordinarily the way things went with fifth metacarpal fractures. 'It's the commonest injury. You always know. That's why they call it the boxer's fracture. When you ask them, people always say they fell. But if you fall, you go like this' – she spread her fingers out – 'and break your fingers – or your wrist. It's a FOOSH, isn't it? Not the side of your hand.'

'What is this?' said the consultant a moment later, holding up a file. 'I've seen this chappie already.'

'You've got the wrong one, hon,' said the nurse. 'Need to learn to read.'

In the anatomy lab, we were still inside the chest. We took Mr Smith's lungs out. They were grey and speckled with soot, bigger than the hole we had made to squeeze them through, and well anchored. At last we wrenched them out and sat them on his stomach. Now we could see the heart, with the aorta plugged into the top (in anatomical drawings it looks like the funnels outside the Pompidou Centre). Or at least that was what you could see on the lecturer's cadaver. In our cadaver everything was squashed and covered in a black felt that came out in pieces: blood. At his death something, in the heart or in one of the heart's great vessels, must have burst, filling his chest cavity with dried clots.

Orientation is key in anatomy, said one of the demonstrators. 'You'll find it easier if you're the sort of person who always knows where north is.' After this I often wondered where north was; it had never concerned me before. It didn't seem immediately obvious. Anatomy took a geographical view of the body. It divided the abdomen into four quadrants, and as soon as I'd learnt the names of these, the four squares became nine. It sliced humans through different planes – coronal, sagittal, transverse. It had its own terminology to indicate where everything was. Towards the midline was medial; away from the midline was lateral; towards the head was coronal; towards the feet was caudal. The back or upper side of anything was the dorsum, the front or underside the ventral surface.

This was fine, except that humans, unlike maps, move about and can rotate through space. So all references were derived from a figure in a fixed posture, the so-called anatomical position: a person standing with his arms at his sides, palms facing to the front, legs together, as though a corpse had been stood upright. The back or top of your hand was the dorsum, as was the top of your foot. 'It will always be called the back, even when it moves to the front,' said the lecturer. My neighbour turned his hands palms up then palms down then palms up again with the help of his scaphoid. My brain felt as though it was doing something similar.

As a GP, I rarely thought about the attachments any more, but I still needed anatomy. It was useful for diagnosis, but also for explanation. Sometimes patients looked up their pain on the internet and found a picture of a structure that appeared to be in the right place – an ovary, a kidney, a rib – and formed a suspicion that was hard to dislodge. Being able to offer certainty was useful. That is not where your pancreas is, I said. That is not your scaphoid. About once a year someone came in with the conviction that their sternal angle was a tumour on their chest wall. This was my best consultation. It is normal, I said, with a conviction I rarely felt otherwise. It is your *normal bone*. I didn't know what caused people to notice things they'd never noticed before, but

I did know that attention amplified – it made lumps bigger. Sometimes I pulled up a Netter drawing on the internet, to help me explain the anatomy better, and in doing so enacted one of his early illustrations, turning an anxious clutch of symptoms into a diagram with a learning point.

In GP you also had to bear in mind the other pictures the patient had of himself: his reflection, his outline, his sense of who he was. Medicine could harm these, and it was easy to forget this in our focus on bones and organs and meat. Sometimes when operations fixed the problem but damaged the patient's picture of himself, the picture took longer to mend than the wound. It took time for patients to accept added structures – stomas, artificial limbs – if they ever did. Illness introduced vulnerability, which could affect the patient's confidence and sometimes even their balance, so that they started falling over even though their legs worked exactly as before. Visible complaints obliterated every other aspect of a person: all they saw was their irregular skin or their patchy hair. Many people seemed to feel that their bodies were incorrectly matched to their selves. Women felt they were men, teenagers that they were adults, and the elderly didn't feel old; they repudiated this body with its failing hearing and its spindly legs. 'It's not me,' patients said. 'I don't recognise myself.'

Only the profoundly ill could not recognise their own faces. When the time came for us to dissect our cadaver's face in the anatomy lab, the professor acknowledged that it was special. 'You may find it less emotive than you expect, but even so, this is an emotive area,' she said. But uncovering Mr Smith's face for the first time was anticlimactic. Standing near his feet, I looked up at him from under his chin: a pointed beard, a sharp nose, lips set like an effigy on a medieval tomb.

As we hammered down into his brow, the bone splintered. The

softness beneath was the periorbital fat, which had to be picked out with tweezers, like extracting the meat from a crab. The tools grew smaller and sharper. 'Please be careful: we're giving you brain knives today,' said the professor. You had to hit the facial bones hard with a little metal hammer to get them to crack. The head bounced on the table. Putting a hand out to hold it in place, I felt an ear through the muslin.

In class we learnt about the skull. Each bone had its own personality. The sphenoid was a lacy butterfly shape; the ethmoid a slab full of bubbles, like a chunk of Aero, a solid that felt like a space. 'I can't believe I'm holding a sinus,' one of the students said. On the train home after class I read my photographic anatomy book. I stared at a coronal view of a human face. The cadaveric section was as full of holes as a slice of Emmenthal; the corresponding CT image looked like a doily. There is so much empty space behind the face. The man in the seat next to me was reading my book too. 'It looks like *The Scream*,' he said.

Perhaps this was why the head seemed perversely less human than the rest of the cadaver. We had spent so long on the body that we felt we would be able to identify our cadaver's heart, should it somehow get separated from the rest of him. The next time we pulled off the covers, we found the face had been peeled by the plastics trainees. They had left skin in islands around the eyes, lips and ears, which added a kind of personality while taking actual personhood even further away.

I learnt the muscles of facial expression on my elective placement, which was in a government hospital in Mumbai in India. The doctor supervising me had about a hundred and fifty patients to look after and he did everything quickly. On ward rounds he would climb over the beds, which were packed together, rather than take a longer route. The patients lay still as he scrambled over them. Once, we had a ten-minute lunch in the café opposite the hospital, and he started a tutorial as we walked across and continued as we ate. He pulled a face for each muscle as he explained it. The 'frowning muscle', corrugator supercilii; the 'blow out your cheeks muscle', buccinator; the 'flare your nostrils muscle', nasalis. He shovelled in his daal. 'Muscles of mastication,' he said, chewing. 'Completely different nerve.' Another time, at the end of a ward round, he called me over and drew the facial nerve in my notebook. 'It's my favourite nerve,' he said, looking at his drawing. Where had I got the idea that nerves were not tangible physical structures? Was it because my primary school teacher had called them invisible wires as opposed to skin and blood, which you could see? Listening to the registrar was like accompanying someone on a tour of his neighbourhood; he pointed out each branch as though indicating the house of a friend. 'And this is the secret branch,' I thought he'd said. Afterwards, looking at Netter, I realised he'd said 'secreting'.

I now knew that each body part had a label. I had once shared with romantic fiction the belief that the body is studded with places too esoteric for anyone to have named – the hollow above the collarbone, the dimple behind the knee, the dip above his manly lips, etc. Soon I discovered everything had been identified. The supraclavicular fossa, the popliteal fossa, the philtrum: there was no fold or knobble too minor for categorisation. I still encountered new words. An ENT doctor teaching me examination skills had me look in his ear with the otoscope. 'Can you see the tympanic membrane?' he asked – the disc of skin that separates the ear canal from the middle ear: it looks like a piece of clingfilm stretched over a bowl of leftovers. Behind the membrane I could see a spindly bone like a chicken leg: the handle of the malleus, the first of the three tiny middle ear bones. I said that I could. 'Can you see the umbo?' This, it turned out, was the most concave point of the tympanic membrane. I did not need this word ever again, which of course meant I never forgot it.

The Dead

There is nothing more dead than a medical cadaver, who has passed into a place where their personhood is absolutely embodied – scrutinised, noticed, remarked on – but also absolutely absent, so that you can batter away at their face with a hammer. A medical cadaver doesn't seem dead in the same way as the patients I met who had died.

Before I started medical school, I had seen a dead person only once. I was about nine years old, standing with my middle brother by the hedge that separated our house from our neighbour's, waiting for our mother. She came out, we set off, and there was our neighbour lying across his front steps. In my memory he had a bedspread laid over him, though in fact this was probably put there later – perhaps by my mother. 'What is the first thing people do when they witness a collapse?' asked the instructor on my first basic life support course. 'Find a blanket,' he said. 'Or a chair. We have noticed that chairs play an important role in the public's response to emergencies.'

If we children found a dead animal or bird in the street, we would squat down to look. There seemed to be more dead creatures about in the 1980s, or perhaps I was just closer to the pavement.

Pigeons, blackbirds, mice. We might poke the corpse with a stick or a leaf to try to turn it over (you didn't want to touch dead things with your hands), a junior autopsy. But a dead human was very different. Our neighbour had no fur, he wasn't squashed, you couldn't see his bones, and we'd only glimpsed him before my mother had told us to go back behind the hedge. But his body laid across the steps was clearly abandoned. No one in life lies face down on a path – not in a public place, or even at home.

When I started work in hospital, I'd look round a curtain rather than a hedge, but I found I sometimes knew when a patient had, as the nurses put it, 'gone'. The dead person would be lying in bed just like any other patient, but she wouldn't be holding her head right, or her hands, and it is amazing how quickly I would realise that she wasn't breathing, given that I never consciously noted that people were breathing but rather assumed that they were. Although perhaps the ability to spot whether someone is breathing or not is something I've learnt along the way without really noticing. The more we learnt, the more we forgot what we hadn't known.

There were two kinds of death in hospital: irreversible, and potentially reversible. If you came upon the patient moments after he'd died, or if you witnessed his collapse, or realised he'd only just stopped breathing, you had a small chance of bringing him back (about one in ten for a cardiac arrest occurring outside hospital, about two in ten if the arrest happened inside hospital). The patient had to be very newly dead for cardiopulmonary resuscitation to have a chance of working. Every year, all the clinical staff did the basic life support course. BLS taught the two basic components of resuscitation: CPR, which is chest compressions and rescue breaths; and how to use a defibrillator. On my first course, one of the F1s worried about starting CPR. Was there a risk that she might make things worse? 'Put it this way,' said the trainer. 'The patient is dead. So anything that happens after that is an improvement.' The floor was covered in pink mannequin torsos, each with its mouth open in a slight half-smile. 'My Resus Annies,' the instructor said. 'All Resus Annies have the same face, based on the death mask of a woman who drowned in the Seine in the nineteenth century. See what can happen when you don't know BLS!'

Death inside hospital is not like death outside. Hospital is a place where death is expected, to a certain extent – it's always a possibility. Deaths inside hospital felt like redundancy, a thing that could happen to anyone but usually happened to someone else, the news passed about quietly. My GP patients sometimes refused to go to hospital at all, citing someone they'd known who never came out. In hospital, arriving to review the patient in bed 5c, I found he was no longer there. The curtains were pulled back, the sheets stripped from the blue rubber mattress. 'He's gone to Rose Cottage,' said the nurse. In some hospitals this meant death, wherever that is – in others, the morgue.

If you were needed for resuscitation, the hospital put out a crash call. Other times the nurses needed a doctor to come and verify a patient who was irreversibly dead. If you didn't go right away, you would get bleeped repeatedly: the patient couldn't be moved to the morgue until his death had been verified, which meant his bed was tied up. Death had to be confirmed and documented in the notes by a specified healthcare professional, which in hospital was frequently a doctor. Before we became blasé – which took about a week – the F1s agreed that this job was unappealing. The thought of a dead patient was unsettling, but so was the fantastic possibility that the nurses might have got it wrong. What if the dead person was not dead after all, *and woke up in the middle of you verifying them?*

To verify the dead, I carried out the same steps each time. I put my stethoscope on the dead person's chest and listened for heart sounds or breath sounds for a number of minutes. (The Royal Colleges specify auscultating for at least one minute, repeated at intervals over a period of five minutes. Five minutes in which nothing happens is a long time.) At the same time, I felt the patient's neck for a pulse. Then I lifted his eyelids, shone a torch into his eyes and looked to see if his pupils dilated. None of these things happened, so I wrote in the notes the phrases that soon became ordinary:

> Asked to verify death.
>> No signs of life.
>> Pupils fixed and dilated.
>> No carotid pulse.
>> Auscultated for heart sounds for one minute: no heart sounds.
>> Auscultated for breath sounds for one minute: no breath sounds.
>> I therefore declare NAME OF PATIENT dead at TIME on DATE.

Some of the doctors added 'RIP'. Once I found a doodle of an angel on the notes of a patient who had died during the night. A little spiral underneath the angel indicated flight.

I found the first deaths unnerving. When I went to palpate the carotid pulse I could feel the pounding of the pulse in my own thumb. The stethoscope rubbed against the patient's hair and converted the sounds into breaths. When I put my fingers on the patient's neck it was sometimes still warm. I wasn't used to listening and looking for things that weren't there: medical school had focused on signs that were present, not absent. It was a relief that the body in the bed was dead and no longer able to judge. The clinical support workers pulled the blinds down, so the rooms were always dim. I would be reluctant to put the light on despite there being no chance of waking the patient. Sitting next to the bed in the half-dark, I would put my stethoscope in my ears and my mobile phone on the bedclothes with the timer on. Then I would wait for enough silence to pass.

The procedure soon became normal. Then one afternoon I was bleeped to the hospital morgue to verify a death, which wasn't normal. How could Mr Smith be in a fridge in the morgue if he'd not yet been verified dead? The technician didn't know, but she was insistent. Mr Smith couldn't be buried or cremated without someone writing I HEREBY DECLARE MR SMITH TO BE DEAD, RIP in his notes. I went to the morgue, which was behind a Portakabin near one of the hospital car parks. Two porters were smoking by the door. 'Here she comes, the angel of death!' one said. I buzzed the intercom.

'I've come to verify Mr Smith,' I told the speaker grille.

'This is the morgue,' a voice replied. 'Everyone in here is dead!'

'But you have a Mr Smith there? Who appears to have slipped through? I've been told he's not been verified yet.'

The technician let me in. There was a wall of metal drawers stacked like a giant filing cabinet. Each drawer had a card inserted into the slot at the front with the name and sex of its inhabitant written on it in black Sharpie: SMITH (M).

I put on some gloves while the technician fetched her key. At this hospital, each drawer held two patients, top to tail, each zipped into an individual body bag. The technician was annoyed; how, she wanted to know, had this person arrived at her morgue before he had been signed off as dead? She opened the drawer, unzipped the body bag, and Mr Smith appeared. He was wearing red pyjamas. His face was white. 'I think he's dead!' I said. The technician didn't think this was funny. She undid the entire zip to check the identity label tied to Mr Smith's big toe. I got ready to listen to his icy chest. 'Is that clock right?' I asked. 'Not been right for five years,' she said. 'Is there somewhere I can balance this?' I asked, holding out my phone.

There were fewer deaths needing confirmation once I became a GP, as fewer people die at home – and they often die at night, when the out-of-hours GPs and paramedics are working; they would then do the verification. But verification was only the first step in the paperwork needed by the dead. Once a person has been confirmed to be dead they need a death certificate, or medical certificate of cause of death, which is filled out by a doctor. The MCCD states the patient's name and address, their birth date and death date, the place of death, and the cause. You write the same information in the margin, which remains behind like a chequebook stub after you've torn out the certificate, making a little flicker-book of recent deaths. I liked reading these, in the same way as I liked reading gravestones. Perhaps my career change was appropriate after all. Death certificates are grandly formal and oversized, like charity presentation cheques. I felt I was defacing them by writing on them in biro; they demand a quill.

Even though death has already occurred, and so nothing can get any worse, the death certificate is always urgent. Without the MCCD, the patient's family is stuck. They can't organise a funeral or a burial or a cremation – the dead person is stuck in passport control. But death certificates also matter to society, as they record the cause of death, which is essential information. The cause of death drives research and healthcare. It facilitates the identification of industrial malpractice, asbestos poisoning, surgical or medical mistakes.

We had a lecture on how to fill in the MCCD at medical school. It transpired that establishing a cause of death is not always straightforward or obvious (England and Wales have started to use specifically trained doctors called medical examiners to assist with this task). As a patient's son once asked me, 'I know he had cancer, but how did he *actually* die?' His father had had lung cancer for months; how did this go from being an illness he endured to one that killed him?

The death certificate required both a cause of death and any contributing and underlying causes. In theory, you could take this exercise all the way back to birth. 'Was born, which led to ageing, which led to decline of cellular regeneration, which led to gene transcription errors, which were aggravated by smoking, which led to mutation, which led to cancer of the lung, which messed up the lung's maintenance systems, which led to pneumonia, which eventually filled all the airways with pus and dead cells so that not enough oxygen could get through, which led to respiratory failure.' But although the MCCD respects (and requires) chains of events, it only has four lines to fill (you didn't have to fill all of them). Documenting for this lung cancer death was relatively straightforward.

I *(a) Disease or condition leading directly to death*
Bronchopneumonia

(b) Other disease or condition, if any, leading to I(a)
Adenocarcinoma of left main bronchus

(c) Other disease or condition, if any, leading to I(b)
Cigarette smoker

II *Other disease or conditions* CONTRIBUTING TO THE DEATH *but not related to the disease or condition causing it.* Hypertension, diabetes mellitus

But sometimes it was harder to ascertain the precise cause of death. Mrs Smith, eighty-six years old, with heart disease, type 2 diabetes, high blood pressure, high cholesterol, thyroid insufficiency, mild kidney failure and a past history of mini stroke – a fairly normal collection of conditions for an elderly person – went 'off legs', as the hospital slang has it, and died twenty-four hours later. Pneumonia causing sepsis? A stroke? Kidney failure? You could not write 'off legs'. 'Old age' as a cause of death was restricted to patients who were really old – certainly over eighty, and most often in their nineties – where you could be sure that nothing else at all was going on. It was hard to feel this certainty. Sometimes, if the death was inexplicable, or if the patient hadn't been seen by a doctor within a fortnight of her death – that is, no doctor had 'attended the deceased during their last illness', as the government guidance expresses it – you would have to report the death to the coroner.

We never learnt how to do this at medical school. My first encounter with the coroner's office occurred when I was a GP trainee. One evening, one of our patients died at home. There was nothing suspicious about the death, but the cause wasn't obvious. I asked reception for the MCCD book and carried it through to my trainer's consulting room, to ask her what I should do. 'He had so many things wrong with him,' I said. I hoped my trainer would reply with a list numbered I(a), I(b) and I(c). Instead she told me to phone the coroner. 'Good learning opportunity!' she said. I went back to my room and rang the coroner's number from the phone list on the wall. 'May I speak to the coroner, please?' I said. 'Hello, this is Sharon, how can I help?' said the phone. 'Are you the coroner?' I said. 'No, I'm Sharon.' I explained that a patient had died and I wasn't sure what to put on the death certificate. Sharon told me to ring her back once I had more information. I read through the notes again and then rang back. 'Hello, this is Jack,' said the phone. 'Is Sharon there, please?' I said. 'She's tied up right now I'm afraid,' said Jack. 'Are you the coroner?' I asked. 'No, I'm Jack.' Jack agreed with my suggested cause of death and said I could fill in the MCCD now. I told my trainer I'd solved the problem. 'You didn't think you would speak to the *actual* coroner?' she said.

Most bodies in Britain are cremated rather than buried. 'Shortage of space,' a GP told us. Cremation had its own set of paperwork, which was in many ways more onerous than the MCCD. The forms we needed to fill in as doctors were the Part Four and the Part Five. Part Four was completed by the last doctor to see the patient before death. You had to write a paragraph explaining how the death had come about – this was more of a detailed story than the numbered list of the MCCD. You stated that you had viewed the body, that it was the right body, and testified that there was nothing dubious about the death. You also had to guarantee that there were no devices attached to the body that might explode in the furnace, such as a pacemaker; to do this you needed to run your hand over the corpse's chest, checking there was no matchbox-sized lump. Once you had completed the Part Four, you needed to find a different doctor to fill out the Part Five, a doctor who knew neither your patient nor yourself who would then be able to act as an impartial witness.

I hadn't been at my new practice for long when I had a phone call from a GP at a different practice asking me to do a Part Five. She introduced herself, explained her patient's death to me, and gave me the number of the district nurse so I could verify the story. I rang the district nurse, who told me the same things. Talking to a stranger about the death of a stranger is dislocating. I didn't like doing it, although phoning a nurse was better than the times when I had to call a family and quiz them about their relative's death. The nurse described Mrs Smith's decline and I wrote notes on a scrap of paper and saw Mrs Smith had been born in the same month and year as me. I felt she wasn't very old, and also I now felt older.

To fill Mrs Smith's Part Five I needed to go to the undertakers. I was always happy to go to the undertakers. A patient in a funeral home was a patient safe from harm, and so I felt a flush of relaxation whenever I opened the quiet doors (all the doors opened quietly). The staff were always friendly, and frequently chatty. The week before, I'd visited a different undertakers to fill a Part Four for one of my own patients. While I waited for a funeral operative to bring me the paperwork, I talked to one of the pallbearers. He was a man in his seventies; he'd been doing the job for fifty years. All the coffins used to be made of oak, he told me, but they were lighter now. 'Although they can still be heavy, if you get a heavy deceased. One at each end and three on each side. It's not the shoulder bit, it's the lift that's hard.'

'That one would be easier, wouldn't it? Wicker?' I asked. There was a woven coffin waiting on a table. 'They can *creak*,' said the pallbearer, wrinkling his nose.

'It's not wicker, it's water hyacinth,' said the operative, coming in with the keys to the fridge. 'Like a laundry basket. Expensive, those are.' She went over to the fridge and opened the door and pulled out the shelf holding the body I'd come to view that day. The runners caught, and it stalled for a moment. 'I know you want out, my love, but it's not time yet,' she said. She turned to me.

'He's one of my tallest. Look how tall he is!' she whispered.

'Why are you whispering?' I asked. 'I don't think he can hear you.'

'I don't know,' she whispered. 'I always think it's best in here.'

I went to do the Part Five for Mrs Smith at the end of my morning surgery. I didn't know this undertakers and rang them for directions, and the woman who answered the phone explained they were located in a graveyard, which was helpful for navigation. Funeral homes are so discreet that I often drove past them, only registering the velvet curtains and urns when it was too late to stop, so that my thoughts about dead people are fused to panicky memories of entrapment in one-way systems.

At the unfamiliar undertakers a funeral operative in a suit showed me into an empty front room. The carpet was so thick it felt spongy. She gave me the completed Part Four to read, and a blank Part Five to fill in once I'd read the Part Four and viewed the body. Then she withdrew, as though giving me space to grieve. I read the Part Four GP's neat handwriting. 'The progression of her motor neurone disease was inexorable. Eventually the decision was taken to transition to palliative care and a syringe driver was started for symptom control.' The operative hadn't come back. I looked at the samples of headstone stone, which had been hung in shiny dominos on the wall. I didn't fancy any of them for myself and wondered about alternatives. Perhaps wicker. I read a price list, which had been mounted in a golden frame.

Motorised hearse only: £419

Motorised hearse with one limo: £500

Horse-drawn hearse including a motorised hearse:

  Set of two horses – black £1185

  Set of two horses – white £1290

I wondered why white horses cost more. Rarer? Harder to keep clean? You could have a 'Memory Bear' for £35; for an additional fifteen pounds it could wear a pink, blue or white ribbon.

The operative was back. 'Do you want to see her now?' she said. 'I'll get my colleague.' She held open a door for me and I went through. Now the floor was uncarpeted and shiny, and the light was as bright as a fridge. It was like going into the stockroom you glimpse through the plastic strips in the supermarket. 'Do you want gloves?' asked the backstage operative, who was dressed in a plastic boiler suit.

There was a trolley in the middle of the room with a body bag on it; they'd got the patient out ready. The woman in the boiler suit unzipped the bag and I saw Mrs Smith. I looked for a moment, then turned away to take off my gloves and wash my hands, even though I hadn't touched anything. 'OK?' said the operative. 'She's not very old, is she,' I said. 'She's the same age as me.' 'Poor lady' said the operative. Back in the carpeted room, I completed the Part Five. Under EXAMINATION CARRIED OUT OF THE BODY I wrote the usual formula: 'External'.

A few days later I found the autopsy report from one of my own patients in my tray at work. Patients didn't usually have autopsies, and a report was a rare thing to read. All of our examinations were external. The front sheet explained that this was 'The details of your patient's final outcome'. Still my patient, even in death. My patient's heart weighed 585g, his liver 1425g, his brain 1370g (I did not know until this moment that the liver was heavier than the brain), his thyroid – a source of anxiety while he had lived – 43g. Over several appointments, we had increased Mr Smith's thyroxine medication, then lowered it back down, trying to balance his blood test results so that he was neither over- nor under-replaced. It was like taking a weight off a scale, watching them equilibrate to not quite level, and then putting the weight back on. At several points I had wondered at the utility of what we were doing, and I had discussed this with Mr Smith. There is sometimes limited gain in trying to get the numbers to come out exactly right. But he was keen to keep trying. He kept a notebook of his results, his blood pressures, his cholesterol readings, his thyroid tests, and he had also found an app that could turn his numbers into graphs, which forced me to recalibrate my own internal scales each time I looked at them, as the tiny numerical trends looked hugely significant when pictured as three-dimensional towers. Total cholesterol 5.5 versus total cholesterol 5.8; what did this even mean, for Mr Smith, or his blood vessels, or his chances of life or death? It seemed unfair that he of all patients should end up needing a post-mortem to tell us the cause of his death. Although I thought he might have liked the detail – there is nothing ambivalent about a pathology report. It is the only way to establish with certainty the exact cause of death. Everything matters, everything is given weight: everything is in fact weighed. 'The lungs are heavy.' I didn't know the implications of this. 'The larynx is unremarkable.' Medical speech: always looking for the remarkable. Still no cause of death. 'On opening the main bronchi some fragments of food material were present on both sides.' It shouldn't be – food should go into your oesophagus, not your lungs – but this information didn't mean much to me without context. I had only cut up one lung in my life; for all I know lungs are usually flecked with morsels of food. 'On removing the brain there was evidence of haemorrhage around the foramina.' So he had had a stroke, an event he had feared, although he had also told me that no cause of death would be too bad 'if it kills me instantly'. The autopsy didn't reveal whether it had done this or not.

Dying

We are not used to death and we are not used to dying either. It used to be more familiar – people were able to read the signs. But now even doctors can be uncertain, and we get anxious about letting people know what is happening. In medical school they taught us what not to say. Giving a prognosis was generally a bad idea: if pushed, you needed to speak of a matter of months, weeks or days. 'If you tell a patient he has six weeks to live he will inevitably go and win a triathlon,' said the lecturer.

Forecasting death was difficult. Sometimes the patient or his family didn't want to know, but you needed them to know so you could arrange for medicines to be delivered and the palliative care team to become involved. Or the family lived expensively far away and wanted exact guarantees about when to book flights home. 'I guess I'll have to come back *again*,' a patient's daughter said as we stood over her mother, who had spurned my suggestion of days and drifted back into weeks. I once sat at a bedside as a patient's wife asked the senior partner how long her husband had got to live. He replied, 'How long is a piece of string?'

One practice gave us a scoring system to help us work out what was going on. You scored the patient based on prognostic signs:

had he taken to his bed? Was he still eating and drinking? Passing urine? Conscious? The sums converted into a green, amber or red code that approximated to weeks, days or hours. When you reached days or hours you needed to think about the end, specifically about doing the administration for the end. You had to talk to the patient and their family about what was happening, and what might happen next. You needed to discuss and sign a Do Not Attempt Resuscitation form, if resuscitation wasn't going to work, to save the patient from an assaulting, unpeaceful death. You needed to prescribe the end-of-life drugs – opioids, sedatives, medicines to help with anxiety and dry up congested breathing – and make sure that someone was able to get the medicines from the chemist, and that they knew what the drugs were for, and had understood that these medicines are not dangerous if used correctly, to take away pain and fear, rather than to hasten death. You needed to make a note for the out-of-hours teams and the district nurses: as babies are born in the middle of the night, people die at dawn and at the weekends.

John Sassall visited his terminal patients several times a week, or even a day. He was present more than GPs are now, although he could do less. One morning, Berger reports, he visits a woman who is dying of heart failure. 'Downstairs in the parlour the doctor explained the medicines he was leaving. The old woman's wheezing was still audible through the floorboards.' Sassall returns the same evening. 'The room smelt now of sickness: under the dressing-table ... there was an enamel bowl with urine in it, and spit stained a little with blood.' The next morning he comes back once again and the patient dies in front of him, 'quickly, her hands very still'. The doctor goes downstairs to tell her husband. As the husband cries, Sassall stands beside him in silence, but we understand his presence is useful.

We have more medicines and treatments than Sassall did, which can mean death happens more slowly. Sometimes I would go out and find a patient had reached what we called the 'terminal phase', but then I didn't get called back for days. The district nurses and the palliative nurses visited in between. When I did visit, my notes were brief: 'cough worse' or 'very tired now'. They were nothing like the observations recorded in nineteenth-century medical journals, which documented decline in minute detail. I remembered a case study published in the *British Medical Journal* in 1861, of a soldier who had contracted meningitis.

> Worse this morning; passed a restless night; was delirious at times, and gropes about on the bedclothes for some imaginary object; he looks stupid and somnolent; is unable to articulate distinctly or fix his thoughts on any particular subject, but does not appear to have lost the power or sensitivity of his limbs; and the pupils, though staring in a state of unmeaning vacancy, are, however, quite regular, and obedient to the stimulus of light.

The case reports have the precision of autopsy reports, except they describe the dying rather than the dead. There was little effective medicine available for anything. This patient was given a 'low unstimulating diet with beef-tea and lime-juice' and a medicine consisting of 'a mixture of chlorate of potash, chloric aether, paregoric and cardamoms'. A weak opioid – which might have helped the pain – mixed with potassium salts, which are now used in the manufacture of fertiliser and matches. Inefficacy did not impede the doctors in their doctoring: they watched, and recorded, and tinkered, and recorded again. Death comes closer with each paragraph and is noted as calmly as everything else. 'He sank quietly on the morning of the seventh day.'

In the twenty-first century, we are not at the bedside as often, and even when we are, we are not looking as hard. We don't record that our patients are searching the bedclothes for lost imaginary objects. Instead we can offer medicines that work, and interventions that change outcomes. But we can't prevent all death. Sassall's patient's husband knew his wife was dying; he knew she would die whatever the doctor did. Now, families don't always understand what is happening, and if they do, they don't understand how we can be letting it happen. As the body nears death, the patient will often stop eating and drinking. Sometimes relatives want this treated: food and drink as medical treatments – a PEG tube for feeding, intravenous fluids. When Mrs Smith had a stroke and never regained consciousness her son was frantic. She remained alive for another fortnight, unable to move, speak or swallow. Her son wanted someone to insert a drip and give her fluids. 'They are starving her to death!' he said to anyone who walked past. I tried to explain that any fluid we gave intravenously would end up in Mrs Smith's limbs, and likely her lungs. There was a woman on the ward upstairs whose hands looked like balloon animals; her finger pads were wet with exuded IV fluid. When the nurses turned her there were handprints on the sheet. I thought of Mrs Smith's grandson trying to hold her wet hand, and how to explain this to her son without making it a horror story. 'Can I not even give her a drink?' he asked.

Medicine colluded with the belief that we could fix everything, even as we aimed to be honest. I learnt to reassure patients that we could palliate every symptom. But you could not always do so, and even if you could, there might be a period where you struggled to get the doses right, or couldn't find anything that worked without causing another symptom instead. Dying at home had become fashionable again – it was felt to be better than dying in hospital.

The idea of the bed takes an important role in this; the belief is that every patient would naturally prefer her own. But these times were sometimes more manageable in hospital or – better – a hospice, where there were other people about, and the whole trauma didn't fall on the family. I wondered if the guidance about dying at home took into account what home is like for some people, or even what death is like from a non-professional point of view. What were you meant to do with it if you'd never seen it before?

The hospices rescued both doctors and patients. You could see the tension going out of families as soon as the patient was installed in this place where they'd worked out how to deal with every fear, down to having red towels in case of haemorrhage (better camouflage for blood than bleeding into white). There were hospices before the 1960s, but it wasn't until Dame Cicely Saunders founded St Christopher's in Sydenham in 1967 that the hospice movement and the discipline of palliative care took off. Saunders began her career as a nurse, retrained as a social worker, and then retrained again as a doctor: as a colleague described her, she was a one-woman multidisciplinary team. Her palliative medicine was evidence based and scientific, but her motivation seems to have been love. As a social worker at Archway Hospital in the 1940s, she met David Tasma, a Jewish refugee from Warsaw, who was dying from bowel cancer. On a six-bedded hospital ward, the two were never alone together, but that did not prevent them falling in love. When Tasma died, aged forty, at 8.40 p.m. on 25 February 1948 (Saunders recorded the time in her diary), he left her £500 in his will to use for 'a window in your home'. 'It took me nineteen years to build the home around the window,' Saunders recalled. Looking for photographs, I expected stained glass, and was surprised to find a window so ordinary looking it needs a plaque under it to explain its significance.

At the start of medical school most of us knew nothing about hospices. We did not understand this field of medicine that did not try to cure disease. A palliative care registrar explained the concept. Addressing all the patient's needs, not just their medical ones. Controlling all their symptoms, not just their pain. She told us the hospice movement had struggled with its image in the early days, recalling a newspaper story headlined *Abandon Hope All Ye Who Enter Here*.

When I thought of hospices, I imagined a hospital with softer blankets and people using quiet voices. We went to visit the local hospice, a modern building on the outskirts of the city. The first thing I noticed was the gardens, which came right up to the windows in a manner that would not have been tolerated by the hospital. I was sent to interview a man who was dying from motor neurone disease. He puzzled me by not being in bed, and not appearing to be dying. He had a computer mounted on his wheel-chair and he typed by blinking. I leant to look at his screen. 'You look worried. What do you want to know?'

Outside the window, a squirrel was stretched like a rubber band between a tree branch and a bird feeder. 'Little shit', the man typed. I realised he meant the squirrel. Later, one of the specialist nurses took us for a seminar. What had we learnt from our day? I mentioned the squirrel. 'He loves birds, so we put him in the best room for birds,' she said. I could not remember the hospital prior-itising wildlife at any point. It reminded me of a moment in Victor and Rosemary Zorza's book *A Way to Die: Living to the End*. Their 1980 memoir of their daughter Jane's death from cancer became briefly famous, and helped to publicise the hospice movement. Jane is a frustrated patient, and the book does not minimise the difficulties of dying. In her last days, Rosemary sees a rabbit out of the hospice window and Jane asks to be lifted up so that she can see it too. I can't, says her mother, worried she will hurt her daughter. 'Oh, Mum,' Jane says. 'My last rabbit!'

After medical school, I never went to a hospice again, as I now belonged to the hospitals. At the start of my first year, it felt as though the patients died constantly. They didn't really – the hospital's rates were normal, there was no scandal – it was just in comparison to life outside, or to my previous life, where no one usually died at all. 'People die a lot,' I said to one of the other F1s. We were each filling in a hospital palliative pathway booklet. Once a patient had been diagnosed as 'end of life', the hospital applied palliative care theory to try to ensure that each death was a good death, even though it was going to be a hospital death with no access to gardens or birds or rabbits. The booklet prompted us to prescribe drugs and to stop non-essential tests and medications so that the dying person didn't spend his last hours being stabbed with needles or woken up to take unnecessary medication. 'A *lot*,' my colleague agreed.

I rarely went anywhere out of range of my bleep, which functioned as a kind of electronic tag preventing the junior doctors from straying further than the Starbucks halfway down the main road. But one weekday I was off, and I had an urge to explore. I was post-nights, a mental state that felt like being drunk, in which the world outside the hospital sparkled with possibility. At the post-nights team breakfast (or was this supper?), time was inverted in a way that was simultaneously liberating and nauseating. Let's go to Keats's house, I said to R. Did you know he started out as a doctor? R recalled Keats had beautiful handwriting. I knew the house was in Hampstead, not far from where we worked. I don't know why I wanted to go. Perhaps I thought that Keats might be infused into the walls somehow and would be able to explain about death.

At Wentworth Place, in the white morning light, all I could notice was how much we weren't in a hospital. No corridors, no swing doors, no lifts, no laminated signs, no alcohol gel, no operating theatres, no radiology department, no gloves. Keats had been apprenticed to an apothecary from the age of fourteen and had gone on to be a trainee at Guy's Hospital, first as a medical student and then as the equivalent of a house officer. In 1817, at the age of twenty-one, he gave up his surgical training. He moved to the house the following year. Wikipedia said he wrote 'Ode to a Nightingale' under a plum tree in the garden. The walls were painted mint and pink, and the window glass was so clean the sky outside looked like a shiny photograph.

Later that year, R and I went to Rome for a weekend. There were many things to do in Rome, but I made us visit the room by the Spanish Steps where Keats had died from pulmonary tuberculosis. He came to Italy with the painter Joseph Severn, who had been recruited by Keats's friends to accompany him on the trip; Severn had agreed without realising how ill Keats was. Keats was twenty-three, Severn was twenty-seven. I was now thirty-four. I already had ten years of extra time on Keats, with nothing to show for it other than a big toe that no longer flexed after walking miles of corridor each day. When I started limping, one of the F2s took me to see his boss, a consultant foot surgeon. The consultant had a look at the end of his clinic. I wasn't officially there, I wasn't a real patient, and I didn't take off my bleep. I lay down on a trolley and the consultant squeezed my foot. He told me the joint had grown some extra bone to try to protect itself, and this bone was interfering with my toe's ability to bend. I tried not to extrapolate anything about the rest of my life from this. It was hallux rigidus, which seemed a nineteenth-century sort of a diagnosis.

The hope was that the Italian climate would make Keats better, but he was unwell on the voyage over, and worse when they arrived in Rome. He knew how sick he was. 'Keats sees all this,' Severn wrote in a letter home, 'his knowledge of anatomy makes it tenfold worse at every change.'

Severn became Keats's nurse. His letters explain his domestic struggles. 'For Three weeks I have never left him. I have sat up at night. I have read to him nearly all day and even in the night. I light the fire, make his breakfast and sometimes am obliged to cook, make his bed and even sweep the room. [. . .] My kettle falls over on the burning sticks – no stove – Keats calling me to be with him, the fire catching my hands and the door bell ringing.'

It took Keats three months to die. On his last day, Severn sketched him, a drawing of Keats's face and head resting on his pillow, like one of Netter's anatomy watercolours, an image float-ing in white space. Although Severn described 'his hair lank with sweat', in this sketch he is beautiful. 'Everything in his room is condemned to be burned even to paper on the walls,' Severn wrote after the death: the Italian authorities decreed this, a futile effort to control the spread of tuberculosis. He wrote down Keats's last words, spoken on the afternoon of 23 February 1821. 'Severn – I – lift me up – I am dying – I shall die easy – don't be frightened – be firm, and thank God it has come!' He died a few hours later.

As a GP, I often went into dying people's houses. Nothing under-lined my freedom like these visits. I was not housebound. I was not unwell. I was not nursing a dying man while doing the housework and staying cheerful. In my first registrar job, one of the patients died at home from the lung disease COPD. He had been ill for a long time, and bed-bound for more than a year; he had a hospital bed in his sitting room, where he now lived. The event of his day was a packet of Hula Hoops, which he would suck, one by one, after lunch, as chewing made him breathless. He only sat up for a bed-wash, or to use the commode, which was tucked in like a spare chair at the end of the bed. His wife had become his nurse. She anticipated his every need; she knew more than any of us about his oxygen equipment and his bed sores. Her life was also reduced to the sitting room, as he couldn't be left alone even for ten minutes in case he choked. The house was pristine, the carpet patterned with vacuum cleaner stripes like a bowling green. My visits left footprints in the pile, although I took my shoes off on the doormat each time, which upset her, as she didn't feel the doctor should be taking off her shoes. A sitter came for two hours, one morning a week, to allow her to go to the supermarket; otherwise, husband and wife spent every day and night together. He went from diag-nosed with dying to actually dying very slowly, one symptom at a time. A stubborn and conscientious man, a retired miner, it was as though he was determined to work through the whole check-list of symptoms and leave nothing out. So he stopped eating, then stopped drinking, then became confused, then drowsy, then developed an odd breathing pattern. Each time, she phoned. 'I am just checking this is OK,' she would say, 'I don't want to cause any bother,' but it was clear she wanted someone to come and see and confirm that this was OK, whatever that meant in this context – of course she did. I tried to go and visit each time, in the gap in the middle of the day that was allocated for visiting, or squeezed in at the end. Dying hours between midday and two, or six and nine. There was nothing for me to do each time but reassure them: this is normal. I tried to think of Sassall, who was necessary even when he did nothing. I offered the patient something for anxiety, some lorazepam, but he wouldn't take it. We agreed he would suck a Polo when the breathlessness ramped up, to add mint flavouring to the inhaled air, a make-believe that it was as fresh and copious as it had been when he was a footballing twenty-year-old. It was easy for me to say 'This is normal', as I got back into my car after twenty minutes holding hands with an angry asphyxiating patient, my shoes soaked from walking across the long grass verge outside their house – no longer mowed short like its neighbours – Radio Two on for its blandness, a woman telling the presenter that she was disgusted. I was alive, this was life, not very exciting, but even my wet feet were proof of my freedom to leave places, my house, their house.

Their road was around the corner from the house where my first dying patient had lived, another retired miner. He died in a similarly pristine lounge, but his death came only a month after receiving a cancer diagnosis, and with 'no warning', as his wife said – that is, they'd had the warning of the diagnosis, but he had seemed quite well if suddenly frail. The next thing that happened was he went to bed for a day, stopped eating, drinking or urinating, and died that night. A block away there was a woman with terminal heart failure, whose bubbling breathing I could always hear as soon as I came into her sitting room, like a filter in a fish tank. I didn't know this part of the city in any way other than as a place where sick people lived. All the well people, in the houses in between, were irrelevant; my eye looked for the plague crosses on the doors. I told the medical students, when I took them out with me in my car for visits, 'That's where Mr Smith lives, he is dying of pulmonary fibrosis. And that's Mrs Smith's house, she has end-stage heart failure.' Their faces controlled, I could imagine what they were thinking: morbid job, driving around bothering dying people, I would like to go back to the hospital where we keep people *alive* – or failing that, at least they die in a thunderclap of blood and shouting and people running about.

But I had been learning that dying took as long as it needed to take, even in hospital. On my last hospital rotation I had helped to look after Miss Smith after she'd been moved to a side room, the privilege reserved for the dying. She was forty-one years old. 'A career girl, and an only,' the Macmillan nurse said, meaning her parents' only child. 'Such a beautiful family.' Her aunt brought in a basket of fruit for the nurses, lined with tissue and heaped with pears and apples and a centrepiece pineapple with a pink ribbon tied like a hairband around its tuft of leaves. They were a cherishing family with nowhere to put their cherishing: even their pineapple was cared for. 'What beautiful fruit,' said Sister. 'She loves fruit,' the dying woman's aunt said. 'All fruit. Especially cherries.' Miss Smith was unconscious for days. Her family came every few hours, gathering in a café near the hospital in between. It had been a year of terrible news. 'Every time they tell us something, it's worse than the time before,' said the aunt. 'We listen to it, we hear it, and then we go to a restaurant. Always a meal. She used to come too, didn't you, my darling?'

Miss Smith had her head propped on a pillow. Her eyes were closed, her face returned to childhood by the swelling around her jaw caused by steroids. The Macmillan nurse stroked her shiny hair. 'See how she is breathing – nothing – then a big breath?' she said.

'Is that good?' asked the aunt, who was sitting on the other side of the bed. No, the nurse shook her head. 'But it's not hurting her. She won't be hurting.'

When the nurses said someone was dying, the person always died not long afterwards. 'Dying people look a little pinched – white – around the nose. And white around the mouth too,' the Macmillan nurse said. 'It's just something you learn to see.' She wasn't using a traffic-light score. This nurse always opened the window after someone died, 'to let the spirit out'. If she couldn't open the window, sealed in as we usually were, she would prop open the door a crack, just enough to show a thin line of the activity outside, the light changing in the corridor as the hospital ordained when was day and when was night. 'You'll be glad to get out of here, my darling,' she told the woman, stroking her forehead. 'Bit of fresh air on your face.'

The Observations

There were five or six pieces of information you needed to know about every patient: the heart rate, the blood pressure, the respiratory rate, the oxygen saturations and the temperature. Together these figures were called 'the observations' (or 'the obs'). In hospital the nurses and clinical support workers took most of the obs and recorded them for the doctors to read. As a GP you had to collect the numbers yourself. The observations helped you identify which patients were doing well and which patients were sick, or becoming sicker.

When the observations confirmed a concern, it felt good, as though your intuition had received a tick. This man is short of breath, I thought as I approached his bed. Correct, I thought, as I looked at his chart: respiration rate 28 (fast), oxygen saturations 92% (a little low). It was helpful if the numbers were bad; you wanted your concerns to sound factual rather than subjective when you phoned your senior about the patient who was pale or drowsy. 'He doesn't look right' was not impressive. 'What's his heart rate?' the registrar would ask. 'What's his blood pressure?'

In GP I encountered the opposite scenario as frequently: a seemingly well person with poor observations. I looked at the person and

I looked at the numbers, and trying to reconcile the two made my face feel tight. Mr Smith had come in about a cough. He was still smiling at my formulaic opening joke when I checked his observations. His temperature was 38.8, so he had a fever. His oxygen saturations were 94%, meaning his oxygen was low. His heart was beating at 115 beats a minute, which is tachycardia. His observations were bad enough to merit admission to hospital, especially as he was also an insulin-injecting diabetic. But he looked as though he was ready to run five miles; if anything, he had grown more relaxed since he came into the room and offloaded his concerns. He had what some of the elderly patients called 'walking pneumonia'.

I considered sending him in to hospital with suspected sepsis. I saw he would be unconvinced, and I knew the hospital would be unimpressed with a patient who neither wanted nor needed to stay in bed. I would be exposing him to unfamiliar germs, and handing over his nicely controlled diabetes to a team who wouldn't understand his insulin regimen as well as he did. Or I could send him home and wait to appear in the newspaper: MAN DIES FROM SEPSIS AFTER GP MISSES SIGNS.

I gave Mr Smith a prescription for antibiotics and made him an appointment to come back for review the next day. I explained the symptoms that would suggest that his condition was worsening, and asked him to call an ambulance if this happened, or the out-of-hours GP service if that happened. Don't *wait* the twenty-four hours until your next appointment if you feel you are getting worse, I said. GPs call this situation 'tolerating uncertainty'. You have to decide what to do even though you may not know exactly what is wrong, how bad it is, or what is going to happen next. It is one of the grand themes of British GP training, along with 'managing risk'. I never got over the way we had tried to encapsulate one of the fundamental difficulties of life in a catchphrase and believed we'd succeeded. Some doctors recited it constantly. 'It's all about *tolerating uncertainty*,' they said, whenever you wondered what you ought to do next. We were meant to tolerate – in fact embrace – what Keats called negative capability: the ability to be in 'uncertainties, Mysteries, doubts, without any irritable reaching after fact & reason'. This differentiated us from hospital doctors, who were all about the irritable reaching – no conclusion without a test or decision without a scan. I found the observations helpful in the mist. Even when the numbers contradicted whatever decision I was making I valued their apparent objectivity, their clarity.

In hospital, the nurses and clinical support workers measured the observations at intervals set by the doctors; we would increase the frequency if the patient became unwell. The CSWs used a tool called a Dinamap, a bleeping blue hatstand on wheels that the doctors were confounded by and so we affected never to know where it was or how to switch it on.

In my first hospital job I was rapidly overwhelmed by the observations: another set of numbers to add to antibiotic doses and cannula gauges. The hospital often measured patients' urine output as another basic observation. The acceptable minimum urine output is half a millilitre (of urine) per kilo (of person) per hour. I found the simple maths of this confounding in the early hours. I would read the urine total from the obs chart, then wait for the number to yield some meaning. Was this a lot? A little? I did not have an innate grasp of quantity. Good doctors have a cook's ease with weights and measures; they know 80 millilitres in an hour is fine without doing any sums. For my first year on the wards I felt the same fear as the innumerate when they shop at a market: is 500 grams of cheese the right amount or have I just purchased the entire wheel?

The other F1 shared my wariness around numbers. Every time anyone told us anything, she would write it down in a notebook in tiny handwriting. One shift, I told her how to calculate an acceptable urine output. The registrar overheard us. 'Very useful,' he said. 'Now, what is the normal range for phosphate?' My colleague looked in her notebook. 'You don't need to know! There is only one thing you need to know, and that is whether someone is sick or not.'

Although they were ill enough to be in hospital, most of the hospital patients were not unwell, most of the time. But some were *sick*. The observations were meant to catch anyone who was *sick*, or getting worse rather than better. The numbers could tell you that things were not right before anyone had realised that things were not right – they were signals.

The obs charts presented a lot of information. We were taught to scan them looking for patterns or pictures that denoted sickness. The blood pressure was usually represented by two chevrons: a ∨ for the systolic, or top number, and a ∧ for the diastolic. In a well person, the number of your systolic blood pressure should be greater than your heart rate. The heart rate was mapped as a dot, like a full stop:

.

On an obs chart this therefore looked like:

∨
.

This was described as 'the seagull crapping' at my seaside medical school. Systolic pressure greater than heart rate: all is well. What you didn't want to see was excrement rising above the seagull – the heart rate accelerating while the blood pressure dropped. This change in physiology, described as 'the cross of death' after the shape it made on the obs graph, meant that the patient had become very unwell.

There were ways to help you digest this information more quickly. The hospitals relied on systems that summed and then scored the different obs, so condensing a person's sickness or wellness into a single number – early warning scores (EWS) or modified early warning scores (MEWS). Early warning scoring systems were developed after research showed that many – if not most – cardiac arrests and other catastrophes that happen in hospital could have been predicted beforehand, from the observations. If you can intervene before the different parameters have veered too far off course, you can sometimes avert disaster. Early warning systems replaced graph interpretation with a score. Now illness, like pain, could be numbered: 'the patient is MEWING a 7'. Different hospitals personalised the names of their scoring systems, so SHEWS, or Sheffield early warning system, etc. The nurse bleeped to tell you that their patient was SHEWING or MEWING or PEWING a 4, and you had to go and review, no scope for prevarication, for interrogating the caller about exactly how ill does your patient look and have you tried sitting them up? In my first week in a new hospital a nurse bleeped to request a medical review as her patient was 'bubbling'. MEWS was invented to abolish the old language of clinical concern: bubbling, gipping, ruttling, 'something not right'.

Outside the charted world, in the community, we didn't have what I suppose would have to be called GPEWS or COMMEWS (although some regions are trying to introduce this now, despite the evidence being poor). In any case, now you had to collect the data before you could work out what it meant. And before you could gather any numbers, you needed equipment.

As a new GP registrar, the practice lent you what you needed. 'Here is the registrar bag,' said the practice manager, handing me a metal briefcase. 'Can you check and let me know if anything is missing?' Reaching into the case I pulled out a packet of condoms. 'That is not meant to be there,' confirmed the practice manager. Once you could manage on ten minutes and were qualified, you needed to buy your own equipment and a bag to put it in. This was generally not leather with a brass clasp, although there was always one registrar in a tweed jacket with a Gladstone bag, asking why we no longer prescribed in Latin. The rest of us chose from: a Samsonite laptop bag; a repurposed baby-changing bag; a polyester 'medical bag' off Amazon; or a suitcase that you could sit on if you preferred not to sit on your patient's sofa (fleas). Later in my GP life, doing visits by bicycle, the main quality I looked for in a bag was compressibility, as I rammed my bag into my basket. Conducting home visits by bike was the only time I felt like a GP that Cronin would have recognised. One day I rode away from a patient's house and almost collided with the postman. 'Don't run over the postman!' he said. 'I haven't been to the doctor in ages and I've got no desire to go.'

'I *am* the doctor, so I guess if I ran you over I would technically have to sort you out,' I said.

'It's a win-win then, isn't it!' We smiled at each other, and I enjoyed the glow of partaking in a period vignette.

The bag was transformed into a doctor's bag by filling it with equipment purchased off medical websites. They stocked everything from alcohol wipes to operating lights. Our needs were modest. Along with a stethoscope and an otoscope you needed an oxygen saturation probe, which told you the patient's heart rate and oxygen level once you'd clicked it onto his finger; a digital thermometer; and a manual or electronic blood pressure machine (or sphygmomanometer, as we never called it, though sometimes we said 'sphyg'). There was no way to work out anyone's breathing rate other than by counting. Officially you did this for sixty seconds, although in reality you were never going to spend an entire precious minute on this. You could count for ten seconds and multiply by six, or fifteen and multiply by four. Or not count at all, if it was a well adult; I suspected most doctors of documenting a best guess. 'The respiratory rate is always 17,' advised a satirical medical website.

The equipment was expensive and fallible. I soon found you could generate any number of temperatures from the same ear by inserting the thermometer at different angles. Once, my thermometer malfunctioned and started generating random but plausible numbers, and it was only when three well-looking patients in a row appeared to have a fever that I realised it had broken. Blood pressures were inaccurate if you used the wrong-sized cuff (most often: a too-small cuff on a too-big arm). Patients had white-coat hypertension – their blood pressure rose in the presence of a doctor – even though no British GP has worn a white coat for years. You could not get an oxygen saturation if the patient was wearing nail varnish or their fingers were cold, and you needed the patient to stay still enough to retain the clip. 'I'm just going to put this on your finger,' I told an elderly patient. 'I'm just going to punch you on the nose,' she said, snatching her hand away and making it into a fist.

On visits, the equipment paraded its vulnerability. The battery ran out in the blood pressure machine. Or the patient's heart was in atrial fibrillation, a rhythm that confuses electronic cuffs into producing unreliable readings. The room was hot or cold, so you didn't trust the thermometer. I was back in the realm of sick or *sick* without any factual information or EWS score to help me. If this was *sick*, I was going to have to go into another room to phone a registrar or an F2 at the hospital to request admission. I had been the F2 receiving this phone call. 'What is the blood pressure?' I don't know. 'What are the sats?' I don't know. In Mrs Smith's front room, the blind had jammed shut. I turned on the light. It had a forty-watt bulb. She was sitting in a recliner chair, blue light flickering over her from the TV. 'I weigh twenty-two stone,' she told me. The electronic blood pressure cuff swelled and then stopped and refused to read. I got my manual one out instead: its cuff was too small to go round her arm. I contemplated joining the two sphygs together and realised I was being ludicrous. The patient's dog licked the sats probe before easing it off with his teeth. Mrs Smith looked jaundiced, but so did my hand when I felt her pulse.

If the numbers alerted me to trouble, I could find myself stuck anyway. I was called for a visit to see an elderly man who lived alone in a sheltered housing block. He didn't come to the door when I rang his bell, but this wasn't unusual. A resident on his way out let me in when I told him I was a doctor; he didn't ask who I was going to visit. I found the patient in the sitting room. The curtains were drawn, but the lamp on the table was on. The patient was sitting up on the sofa, in his pyjamas. He didn't seem too unwell, although he was obviously in pain from the stiff way he turned his head to look at the door, and pyjamas outside the bedroom are not a good sign; nor is a switched-off television. Mr Smith explained that his back hurt and so he had called to ask for a visit. He had been sitting on the sofa, next to the phone, since he'd rung in the middle of the morning. It was now one in the afternoon. Mr Smith looked uncomfortable but not unwell. But when I put the probe on his fingertip to get his oxygen saturations, it read 80%. This seemed impossibly low. I moved it to the other hand – the number still flickered around 80. I counted his pulse:

125. He was looking into my face. 'I need to call an ambulance for you, right now, I'm sorry,' I said. 'I can't put my dressing gown on,' he said, 'my back.'

I phoned 999 from my phone. 'Is he conscious?' said the operator. 'Is he breathing?' The ambulance took twenty-five minutes to come. Mr Smith didn't want to talk. There was nothing I could do: I had no oxygen. I wondered what was making him so unwell – I guessed a leaking aneurysm, or some cancer attacking his bones, or a heart attack that was presenting in an unusual way. His back pain was high up, between his shoulder blades, and tracking round into his right ribs at the front. The pain was so bad when I examined him that tears started to creep down his cheeks, although he didn't make a sound. I stopped my examination. I was adding nothing. I phoned the person he told me was his closest relative, a nephew, and explained that Mr Smith was very unwell and that we were waiting for him to be taken to hospital. Then I went into the bedroom and found a sports bag with a broken zip. I opened a drawer. Folded clothing lay in a single layer – two jumpers, two T-shirts, a vest. I found the jumper he had asked me for, and put it in the bag, along with a carrier bag full of his medicines, which I had found on the coffee table. When I went back to the sitting room Mr Smith's face looked dusky. I was sure he was going to die in front of me. He said he felt sick. I went into the kitchen and opened every cupboard before finding a washing-up bowl in the sink. I tipped out the scourer and took him the bowl. I was helpless. I knew how to do cardiopulmonary resuscitation, but his heart was still beating. I would have to wait until he died before I could do anything. I knew how to treat someone who was this unwell in hospital, but we weren't in hospital; we were in a sitting room with the curtains drawn. He couldn't lie down because of the pain. My fingers were buzzing with adrenaline. I couldn't stop checking my watch. I was counting the minutes until the ambulance, but also counting the minutes until the start of my afternoon surgery: now it was thirty minutes, now twenty minutes until twelve people would be waiting to see me at ten-minute intervals.

The paramedic came into the sitting room, big and bright in his high-vis jacket with his radio. 'This is Mr Smith, and he's about to arrest,' I said. I had sat down next to Mr Smith and we were waiting and sweating together. In the absence of anything else to do I was holding his wrist. His pulse was 140 and weak. This was observation with consequences, and I had no way of changing any of them. All I could do was watch. I had counted as Mr Smith's pulse rose; I hadn't been able to bring myself to repeat the blood pressure, knowing it would barely register; it seemed disgusting to measure a man's observations as he died. Mr Smith had his eyes closed and he was no longer speaking. 'Ah, we'll get you right,' said the paramedic, turning on a canister of portable oxygen. He started his own observations. The numbers showed bigger on the paramedic's rugged equipment, and they were worse. 'He's about to arrest,' he said into his radio. In moments another paramedic came bounding in. Together they took Mr Smith away. In the time called 'peri-arrest' you're in a pause where you feel you have a chance of averting disaster, but in fact you rarely do – if physiology has come to this point, it has a momentum that is very difficult to stop.

Mr Smith's nephew phoned me at the end of afternoon surgery to tell me that he had died half an hour after arriving at the hospital. He had been taken to a resuscitation bay in A&E and had died there shortly afterwards. His heart had stopped, and they had not been able to restart it. The hospital told the nephew that it was probably a ruptured aneurysm. The nephew thanked me for packing the bag – 'It's so important to have your tablets, when you're in – they can never find out what you're on otherwise.'

Breathing was hard to be perfectionist about. To get an accurate respiratory rate, your patient needed to be in a 'resting state' (not have just run up the stairs or become agitated in the wait to see the doctor). We can exert conscious control over our breathing, and so a person who realises you're monitoring them will speed up or slow down. The key to working out the rate was to pay attention without seeming to do so. The teaching I had at medical school was frank in its advocacy of subterfuge, which is now unusual in other contexts. Ordinarily you're not encouraged to deceive your patients, unlike formerly, when deception was fine, in fact was sometimes felt to be the best strategy, with therapeutic benefit – concealing patients' diagnoses from them, for example, in order to preserve hope. One way of counting breaths is to look as though you're taking your patient's pulse – holding their wrist and looking at your watch – while covertly watching the rise and fall of their chest.

I sometimes skipped counting resps as it was difficult and took a long time. On a shift as a paeds F2 at the children's hospital's emergency department, I saw a nine-year-old boy who had been brought in because he was vomiting. He was leaning on his mother, holding a toy bucket into which he retched occasionally. His mother was a small woman in a headscarf and a long cardigan. She didn't speak much English; the boy's twelve-year-old sister had come along to help with translating. Every time the boy retched, his mother rubbed his stomach. He looked tired. He was my eleventh patient that evening, and I had already seen several other children with diarrhoea and vomiting, all from the same part of the city, and all with Bangladeshi parents – I'd even seen another Mohammed, whom the registrar had discharged home.

We are taught to look for patterns. All the children attended the same school. I thought they might be sharing a stomach virus. As it seemed obvious what was wrong, I didn't repeat the obs, but looked at the admission card instead, where the triage nurse had written down everything as it had been when Mohammed arrived. He was tachycardic, but nothing else was wrong on the admission numbers – his oxygen saturations were perhaps slightly low at 96, but not low enough to make me think of danger. His mouth was hanging open and his lips looked dry; I judged him to be dehydrated, probably from vomiting; his mother said he hadn't urinated much since that morning, and he had been vomiting all afternoon. He was complaining of tummy pain and holding his hand over the left side of his abdomen. I listened to his chest, as best I could through the retching, but didn't count his breaths; I looked in his ears and down his throat; I felt his abdomen, which was soft and not tender when I pressed on it. I made a plan for him to be set up with a fluid challenge – a plastic cup of orange squash, to be syringed into his mouth, with a piece of paper for his mother to record how much he'd taken; his sister took the syringe and the paper from me and told her mother the plan. I prescribed some paracetamol, as he had pain and a low fever. I planned to review him in an hour, to see if the fluid had made him any better.

Twenty minutes later, Sister came to the desk where I was sitting writing up the notes. 'Who is looking after Mohammed? You need to see him now.' My heart started to bang. 'He was fine just now?' I said. 'He was vomiting, but he was settled.'

'He's ill. He's gasping, he's got tracheal tug and his sats are 90.'

I realised I knew this information already but had failed to interpret it. I had seen the tracheal tug – the muscles pulling in and down at the base of the child's neck, where he was recruiting extra muscles to help him to breathe – but had thought that it was due to retching, even though the sign didn't fit. Retching is random and irregular; tracheal tug occurs with every breath. My brain had discarded one of the facts because it didn't fit the story.

The nurse had put an oxygen mask on Mohammed and given him ten doses of Ventolin through a plastic spacer tube. He now had a sats probe taped to his finger. His eyes were no longer sleepy but dilated with panic and salbutamol. His mother was quiet; his sister said, 'She wants to know what's wrong.' I listened again to his chest. I could now see the indrawing muscles between his ribs. I also heard what wasn't there. There were no breath sounds at the base of his lung on the left side: reduced air entry. I had forgotten to notice what was absent in my concentration on what was present. The debris of infection was blocking his airways and not allowing air to pass in or out. He had pneumonia. The pain in his abdomen was coming from his chest; his retching was being caused by the infection making him unwell. I requested a chest X-ray and prescribed intravenous antibiotics and oxygen, and scrabbled in the equipment room to get a tray together to put in a cannula. I felt the shame of the misdiagnosis throughout. Years later I felt the same shame when I read about the case of Dr Hadiza Bawa-Garba, a paediatric registrar who was convicted of manslaughter in 2015 after misdiagnosing a six-year-old boy who died of septic shock. She thought the boy had gastroenteritis when he in fact had pneumonia. No nurse or colleague rescued her from her mistake.

Perhaps for similar reasons – not being able to see what is in front of you because you've already decided what it is – I found diagnosing my own children difficult. At the age of two, my son caught the ninth or tenth cold of his life. Like all his colds, it made him wheeze. At eight months he had been admitted to hospital for wheezing, and we'd had to stay in for two days waiting for his oxygen levels to return to normal. As usual when he was ill, he was not upset. When we stood next to people in the post office they leant over his buggy and asked him 'who's a bit snuffly?' It was obvious to anyone that he was working to breathe, but it appeared his body considered this another of the tasks that are required to get on in life, like learning to climb stairs. I knew from reciting to patients that I was meant to 'trust my instincts as a parent' – but my instincts had been perverted by the observations. He wheezed through the night. At three in the morning, holding a torch over him as he heaved and choked, R and I decided we would take him in if he carried on like this. In the morning, he was as energetic as ever. He ate breakfast. He's fine, we decided; we have medicalised him. We'll keep him at home. In the evening he coughed and panted and wheezed again. I sat next to his bed. Occasionally he half opened his eyes. He looked tired. I held my phone in my hand to count his respirations; I had taken his temperature about fourteen times. I was fitting the numbers into the traffic-light guide for sick children, the algorithm GPs use to assess whether children are unwell enough to need to go into hospital. His respirations were 60, his chest was pulling in and out. We went to the hospital.

Arriving at children's A&E, we were sent straight to triage, where H's observations were deranged. I admitted I was a doctor. 'Did you not notice his breathing?' the staff nurse said. She gave him some salbutamol. After a short rest H jumped out of my arms and climbed a pile of foam blocks in the soft-play area. My worry about illness was replaced with worry about fraudulence. He looked frisky. Around us, children lay across their parents' laps, or held injured limbs out in front of themselves.

Forty minutes later, H came to sit down again. They put us in a room on the observation ward. Now he looked pale. The registrar asked for him to be put on a monitor, 'to keep an eye on his heart rate'. I sat in the dark with him on my lap, watching the numbers. Some subconscious pull was making my breathing fall into step with his and I became aware that he was panting. I counted in elephants – sixty a minute, seventy. He felt heavy, and I became aware of a wet patch on my thighs as he sweated, although his forehead felt dry. I pressed the call bell for the nurse; when she came, I explained I was worried by his breathing rate and by his heart rate. He felt hot. She took his temperature, which was 41 degrees. She called the registrar, who put her stethoscope on his chest and lifted it off and put it on again. 'He isn't shifting any air at all! Aren't you a doctor? Why didn't you have a listen?' 'I'm his mother,' I said. It sounded weak.

This time he had pneumonia, and we stayed in for three days, for oxygen and intravenous antibiotics. Time went slowly. One evening, I went into the little side room where the parents of the long-term patients had a fridge for their ready-meals and milk and spreads. They had their own mugs. I felt golden luck that I had no mug, that our child was only temporarily unwell. I immediately regretted my smugness and wondered what punishment would follow.

The day began at six, when the nurse came to do H's obs. It was a hundred years until ten, when the ward round arrived. I would see them through the little window in the door, taking the obs sheet out of its plastic holder, and I would rehearse words in my head, needing to get everything said before they went away again. After that, nothing happened. We walked up and down the corridors, to the toilet and back, to the playroom and back, to look at the lift buttons and back. We walked past a mural on the wall, a top-heavy elephant. He had drooping eyelids and was gesturing with his trunk at a mouse. The mouse stayed out of his reach. Three times a day a meal came. They were as exciting to receive and as disgusting to eat as meals on an aeroplane. They worked for dividing up the day, until it was time for the drip.

The cannula fell out four times during our stay. 'Magic cream!' said the nurse, smearing local anaesthetic onto H's wrist. Then it was time for the side room and a screaming pin-down session. 'I know I'm meant to say he's not usually like this, but I'm afraid he is usually like this,' I said to the nurse as she held his flailing arm. Later, doing a paeds job myself, I would examine a lot of children and put cannulas into some of them. I continued to follow her instructions. 'The first thing to do is to get them sat right.' I showed parents how to angle children on their laps, one arm round here, the other round here, one arm binding the child's arm, the other anchoring his head. Successfully immobilising your child patient was a crucial skill in paediatrics. You can't throw an apple into a moving car, can you?' the paeds F2 said. 'Likewise: you can't look into a moving ear.'

Eight months of my GP training was in the same children's hospital. When I was first bleeped to the ward, I was embarrassed, thinking they would remember me walking up and down the corridor in my pyjamas and not believe I was a doctor. But no one recognised me with a stethoscope round my neck. I roamed the hospital, running up and down the stairs, along the corridors, down to theatres, up to the neurology ward. Every time I saw the elephant, I felt I had escaped. I remembered when my son's observations went wrong in the middle of the night, and how nice it was to see a doctor, and how I'd wanted to help her by sharing lots of information with her, and how she'd wanted to continue with the jobs list that I could see folded and clipped to her bleep.

Before we started paediatrics, the new trainees had to attend a teaching session on paediatric emergencies. The instructor was a consultant in a pink shirt. He flapped his tie at us: it had a pattern of tiny elephants. 'That's in case you didn't realise I'm a paediatrician,' he said. After telling us what a great time we were going to have on the job, he picked up a plastic resuscitation dummy and held it against his chest. He talked to us about what to do when a child becomes suddenly unwell. He explained the untrustworthiness of their observations. Children are generally healthy and fit; their youthful physiology can compensate for and mask deterioration. 'Do not trust the blood pressure,' he said. 'They can keep it going fine until they're basically dead.' The seagull analogy was useless here. 'In fact, don't be doing a blood pressure at all if they look unwell – get on with treatment.' Soon the dummy was on a table and he was kneading its chest vigorously with two stiff fingers, the neonatal version of CPR.

'Ow, poor baby!' one of the trainees said.

'I see you, in your fluffy pink cardigan – you're a fluffy kind of person – hey, so am I, I'm a paediatrician. But you have to do it like this or you might as well not do it at all,' said the trainer. 'And see, I put my other hand on its head, because it makes me feel fatherly. Not really: I do it because resuscitating children makes me feel squeamish and this is my way of coping with that squeamishness.'

We sat in silence. We could hear the traffic outside, and the rubber exhalation of the resuscitation baby and the thud of its head bouncing against the table. One of the first things you learn about CPR is that you never pause – once you've begun, you go on and on until someone says it is time to stop. This is so ingrained that even if it's only a plastic model the trainers often carry on pumping while they're talking.

'You just keep doing it. Over and over. So you don't have to remember it. So your hands know it. So when you're thinking *fuck fuck fuck, what did Dr Smith say?* your hands know what to do. Ah!' He shook the baby gently. 'A sign of life! Stop and reassess! Start again: ABC. After that? Check his numbers.'

The Heart

The most important numbers, the heart rate and blood pressure, are generated by the heart. The heart is the centre of everything. You could afford not to know about other specialties' organs eventually – you didn't have to cultivate a detailed understanding of the eye, or the foot, if you were planning to be a colorectal surgeon. But the heart could not be omitted. It ensured we paid attention by sometimes stopping.

We knew about hearts already. Unlike the pancreas, or the pituitary gland, it was a famous organ. We knew where the heart was. We could feel it beating in our chests and sometimes in our abdomens. We had pulses that accelerated with exams or public exposure. We knew what a heartbeat sounded like. As children, we had put pretend stethoscopes onto adults' chests to hear them say 'Bu-dum bu-dum!' We had watched films where a character is trapped in a dark alley to a soundtrack of amplified BA-BOOM! BA-BOOM! But medical school took these hearts away and started again, at the beginning. We needed to understand that this was an electrical, mechanical pump, and the magic was science.

I knew the heart was not a cut-out shape with two curves at the top, but I still found its appearance surprising when we opened the cadaver's chest. It was larger than I'd expected, about the size of a fist. The heart doesn't just contract and relax, but also twists a little with each beat, generating its own torque, the cardiology professor said. In a tank of water it would propel itself like a squid.

Every cadaver's heart looked slightly different. Ours was fibrous and squashed like a dried fig, from having been starved of blood in its final minutes. The heart of our neighbours' cadaver was huge and round, its muscular walls stretched thin; the patient had died of dilated cardiomyopathy. We passed the heart around. It reminded me of an ocarina, hollow and hard, with the holes where the great vessels had been connected sticking up like mouthpieces. As a GP, years later, I grew used to seeing patients with heart failure. I would guess the diagnosis when Mr Smith told me that his ankles were always swollen and that he felt breathless when he lay in bed. When I listened to his chest I could hear the fluid crackling at the base of his lungs and when I pressed on his legs my fingers left dents. I put my hand on his chest to feel for the apex beat, where the heart can be felt knocking against the surface (this point is lower than you might think, as the apex of the heart is at the bottom: anatomical labels often describe where something was in the embryo, and expect you to remember all the folding and rearranging that takes place before birth). Mr Smith's apex beat was no longer lined up below his nipple, but had moved out sideways as his heart had grown baggier.

The cardiology professor invited one of his colleagues to come and lecture us on physiology. Professor Smith was retired, but too in love with hearts to stop working. He walked up and down the stage of the lecture theatre, forgetting to change his slides. He told us about William Harvey, the famous English physician who worked out how blood circulates round the body in 1628. 'A proportion of patients believed he was my uncle. For the simple reason that I had his portrait hanging in my office, and when people asked about it – asked who he was, I used to say, "He is my uncle."' It was all just plumbing, Professor Smith said, trying to make it easier for us; but I knew he didn't believe this himself, for how often does plumbing generate electrical currents?

After dissecting hearts, we had to learn to listen to them. When I started using a stethoscope, I couldn't hear the right noises. First, I heard nothing at all. I put the stethoscope in my ears and all the sounds in the room switched off as though I'd put in ear plugs. When I put the chest piece on the patient the silence continued. I looked up to see the lecturer miming a twisting movement. I had swivelled the chest piece to the bell side but was listening through the diaphragm. I subsequently learnt to tap the chest piece with my fingers to check which side was on, a gesture I initially performed with drama but which dwindled to a flick as the equipment grew familiar. I already knew not to drape the stethoscope around my neck when I wasn't using it, as to do this would signal obnoxious entitlement. The students observed this rule so conscientiously that when I first wore a stethoscope at the start of F1 I felt as though I'd put on a boa constrictor.

When I laid the chest piece of the stethoscope on the patient's skin there was an immediate cacophony. The noise was even worse if his chest was hairy. The sounds were amazingly various, but they were clearly not heartbeats. I remembered a childhood visit to the Natural History Museum in London. Mum took us into the womb room, a pink cave playing an amplified maternal heartbeat, which aimed to reproduce the experience of being a fetus. I was horrified and fascinated and kept rebirthing myself so I could go in the room again. I had assumed the stethoscope would provide the same immediate surround-sound experience. 'You have to let your ear go inside while you stay outside,' the professor said.

We learnt to move our stethoscopes across the chest in a set routine to listen to each territory of the heart: aortic, pulmonary, Erb's point, tricuspid and mitral. 'All Pigs Eat Too Much,' one of the students said. No one was puzzled by this random remark: we were always avid for a mnemonic. I did not know who Erb was, but I accepted him immediately, as I had Virchow, who had a triad, and Janeway, who owned some lesions. 'The dance of the stethoscope,' the professor said, pirouetting from the diaphragm to the bell to capture low-pitched sounds as he moved over the patient's chest. His free hand held the patient's bare shoulder. The patient was smiling.

The professor had an intimate relationship with each of the heart's sounds. 'The second sound is really *lovely*,' he told us. 'One has to love the second sound.' The fourth heart sound, on the other hand, 'is not a sound. It's an awareness of the ear drum going *in* ... then *out*. No one can hear it these days. Well, maybe my colleague Dr Smith, but no one else.' We nodded; who knew what anyone else could hear? We would step up to Harvey, the school's anatomical simulator, lay on our stethoscopes, frown to indicate listening, then step back with a nod. On Harvey the heart lifted up his rubber skin a little with each pulse, like a drum skin moving, making it easier to cheat.

The textbook description of normal heart sounds was 'lub-dub'. The first and second sounds are different, the professor explained. 'Lub' is the sound of the atrioventricular valves closing. Once the top two chambers, or atria, have finished emptying blood into the bottom two chambers, or ventricles, the valves between them clamp shut in order to prevent blood leaking backwards. 'Dub' occurs after the ventricles have pumped the blood out of the heart and into the big blood vessels. The flaps of the aortic and pulmonary valves are more rigid than those of the atrioventricular valves, so the sound they make is shorter and crisper. The distinction was essential – without knowing which was the first and which was the second heart sound, you couldn't interpret any additional noises. Was this a diastolic murmur, occurring while the heart was filling, or a systolic murmur, occurring as the heart emptied? 'If you can put your index finger between the second heart sound and the murmur, it's not a pan-systolic sound. A pan-systolic sound *wraps around* the second sound,' said the professor.

Once I'd finally got my ear inside and heard a heartbeat, I couldn't stop hearing heartbeats. The heart drowned out the lungs, and I couldn't hear breath sounds any more. My brain tried to force all rhythms – train wheels, music, typing – into lub-dub. At home the ceiling in my bedroom had started to leak, each drop falling on the wooden floor with a click. I tried to decide which drip was the first sound and which the second. I thought how I would annotate the rhythm in the notes. HS 1+2+0, we had learnt to write, which meant we had heard lub, dub, and nothing else; as opposed to HS 1+2+ESM – lub, dub, and an ejection systolic murmur. Some people drew shapes to represent the noises they'd heard: 1◊2, with a diamond to signify the crescendo-decrescendo whoosh of aortic stenosis; or 1□2, with a rectangle to represent the blowing sound of mitral regurgitation, which is the same volume throughout.

I always found listening an effort, but for Smith, it was easy. Sounds seemed to float through him without thought. He was a tall boy who always had headphones around his neck. Even when his headphones weren't on, leaking metallic bits of percussion, he looked as though he was listening to something. 'What can you hear?' asked the cardiology professor, watching Smith as he touched Harvey's chest with his stethoscope. The professor was nearly four times Smith's age, but the top of his head only just reached Smith's shoulders.

Smith pulled the stethoscope out of his ears. 'Lub-dub-dubcha -dubcha-bup-cha-CH-BUP-ch-cha-ch-CH,' he said, moving his head a little as he made the sounds. 'Exactly so,' said the professor, nodding briskly. It was atrial fibrillation (the commonest cardiac arrhythmia), performed in beatbox. 'How about this one?' the professor asked, touching Harvey's controls. Smith nodded, listened, and then said 'lub-dup-*tss!*' Harvey had developed pulmonary regurgitation – the blood was backflowing through his pulmonary valve. 'Quite!' said the professor. 'This is not a "whoosh". It's a "puff" of air. A little blow.' He pursed his lips as though to blow out a candle. They smiled at each other.

One afternoon a friend and I sat in Starbucks, revising for our clinical exams. I had found some recordings of heart murmurs online. We were trying to memorise the abnormal noises in case they gave us a patient with these sounds in their chest. My laptop sat on the table playing lub-dub, lub-dub. My friend had found some lung recordings. We were on our way to soundscaping a complete human being: one of our computers was wheezing and the other had a racing heart. 'The famous medical sense of humour,' said a woman sitting next to us.

As well as listening to the heart, we learnt to feel its transmission, the pulse. I was inclined to pulses as they fitted my romantic concept of a doctor. The venerable names worked for this vision – pulsus paradoxus, pulsus tardus. The act of taking the pulse brought a vision of a bearded gentleman lifting the wrist of a pallid lady lying in a feather bed. A pause; the wrist handed back; a pronouncement. The doctor controls the plot! I knew from nineteenth-century novels that taking the pulse was a vital part of doctoring.

The cardiologists brought in patients with rare signs for us to examine. All the specialties told us to think horses not zebras, and then showed us zebras to lure us in. An actual water-hammer pulse. A man with Quincke's pulse, whose nailbeds flicked from pink to white with each heartbeat. Examining the arterial pulse was such an ancient medical gesture it made you feel more like a doctor each time you did it. Also, it was easy; when you pressed in the right place with your fingers the pulse was there beneath them. It was not the same when I tried to examine the pulses behind the knees. Foot pulses were even worse, and you started out with no dignity even before you'd failed, as you had to crouch down on the floor. I didn't remember anyone in *Middlemarch* having to examine foot pulses.

Once I'd graduated, my surest procedure in hospital involved sampling the radial pulse to collect an arterial blood gas, or ABG. I had seen how cardiology loved to transform one thing into another – sounds into pictures, rhythms into diagrams. An ABG was a practical procedure that converted the sensation of the pulse into actual arterial blood. To take one, you needed to feel for your patient's pulse at the wrist and then remember the exact point where you'd felt the movement. A colleague used to draw a dot with his pen, as though marking where he planned to drill, although if you did this and then stuck your needle through the dot you risked giving the patient a tattoo as well as a scar.

To take the sample, you pushed a small needle in at an almost ninety-degree angle. If you were in the right place arterial blood filled the syringe immediately, nudging the plunger with each heartbeat. Your next job was to find an analysis machine. There were only ever a few in the hospital, situated in the crisis areas – A&E, intensive care. Although ABG syringes contain anticoagulant the blood still wants to clot. As I waited for the lift I would roll the sample between my hands, willing the blood to stay liquid. Often there was a queue at the analyser and everyone looked like they were on a wilderness survival course, twizzling sticks between their palms in the hope of starting a fire. Once you'd given your sample to the machine to drink it was a few minutes before you found out if all was in vain: you'd drawn venous blood by mistake, or picked up an air bubble. At last, the analyser printed out a paper slip that showed the blood levels of oxygen and carbon dioxide (among other things). In my first job we had to tape the slip into the patient's notes and then copy the information out as well, as it transpired that the printer ink was not permanent and faded to invisibility over time. 'You have to do *what*?' said the new F1 when I explained this part of the job.

Changes in the heart's rhythm usually signalled an abnormality. There was the so-called gallop rhythm, where the presence of an extra heart sound causes a 'lub-dub-dub, lub-dub-dub' noise, like a horse's hooves. 'If you're not a horse person, you can think of the word "Ken-tu-cky",' suggested the professor. Or the rhythm could break down completely, into the 'irregularly irregular' chaos of atrial fibrillation, or AF. The 'lub ... d-lub ... dub ... dubdubdub ... lub-d ... lublub' sounds were caused by the atria fibrillating, or 'dithering', as the professor described it, and so filling and emptying in a chaotic fashion.

In hospital we saw patients who had gone into fast AF. They looked pale, breathless and unwell as their hearts pounded along chaotically at a rate that failed to provide any useful blood supply to their organs. In the community I often discovered AF in people who weren't ill. The first time I found it, I doubted it. The patient had come in about a cough. She told me about her Christmas plans while I held her wrist. Her pulse was irregularly irregular, with no pattern in the irregularity, no predictably dropped beats. 'Jazz solo,' as one of our lecturers used to say. It didn't seem possible that the patient didn't know this information herself; how had she become so estranged from her own heartbeat? But we don't notice our own heartbeats, or we would go mad with listening. She didn't believe me even when I had her feel her pulse herself; and then, when she did believe me, she became agitated. Everyone knows the heart is important, so a heart that isn't conforming to the basic rule of rhythm is alarming. I tried to explain. You have a condition that you can't see and may never feel. It is your heart, but it is not usually dangerous to your heart. I then had to explain it might be dangerous to her brain instead. 'You *what*?' said the patient.

In atrial fibrillation, the blood churns and eddies instead of flowing smoothly, which can make the red blood cells cling together instead of sliding past one another. On an echocardiogram this makes a sign that the cardiologists call 'smoke', the invisible flow becoming visible. The eddying cells can form a clot, and the clot can then go up to the brain, causing a stroke. We had to start the atrial fibrillation patients on anticoagulants – blood thinners – to prevent this from happening. 'Rat poison!' said every patient at the mention of warfarin. 'But I'm already on aspirin?' Different kind of clot, I said, as convincingly as a train company referencing different kinds of snow. The novel anticoagulants, or NOACs, were easier to start than warfarin, with its four hundred interactions and its labile blood levels and need for constant monitoring; but unlike with warfarin there was no reversal agent. If you fell, and you bled, you could bleed uncontrollably. If you fell on your head, you could bleed into your brain, another kind of stroke caused by the medication you were taking to try to avoid a stroke.

Through the stethoscope, the chaos rhythm of atrial fibrillation was easy to diagnose. Other heart conditions caused sounds that were harder to interpret. There were clicking and snapping noises, generated by stiffened valves opening or shutting. There were sloshing and rumbling sounds – heart murmurs – caused by the blood changing speed and direction. Sometimes there was a mechanical clunk from a prosthetic valve. At medical school the cardiology lecturers brought in volunteer patients for us to examine. The patients were expert and charming. 'My robot heart!' said an elderly man standing with his shirt open as we filed past his chest. Another man pulled out a fob watch on a chain and offered it to us for timing his pulse. He had brought all his medical notes with him. 'I had a triple in 2001,' he told us. 'See there – it's on the summary sheet at the top.'

Ten years after graduating I was in my consulting room with Mr Smith. He had first come to see me the week before, saying he felt more breathless than usual. When I listened to his chest, I realised he had a heart murmur. I think it's aortic stenosis, I told him, but I can't be sure until you've had an ultrasound scan to look at your heart valves. I was trying to stop myself from saying 'jelly scan of the heart' to explain the echocardiogram. I found the phrase weird and unilluminating, but it was so ingrained that I often said it without realising. I used chevrons <> to type the diamond shape for crescendo-decrescendo in the notes, which was unnecessary – *extra*, the current medical students would have said – but I still liked that a sound could have a shape. Now Mr Smith had come back for a second appointment, to discuss starting some statin medication. He had already consented to be examined again and he did not pay much attention as I went through the medication with him. 'Whatever you say, you're the doctor,' he said. Then he tugged at the front of his shirt and raised his eyebrows at the two medical students sitting silently on their chairs behind me.

'Shall we?'

'Let's,' I said. I remembered Professor Smith standing with his hand on his patient's shoulder, both of them beaming as though they were about to give us a present.

Surgery and Medicines

One weekend I read a newspaper article in which William Boyd, the novelist son of a doctor, discussed the phenomenon of surgeon authors. He talked about the adventure of surgery: cutting into flesh, creating and mending wounds; about lifesaving operations, and bad outcomes, patients maimed or dead. It sounded exciting: I envied the surgeons their stories. I was weeks into medical school before I realised that medicine could be divided in two. There was Surgery, which created surgeons, who performed operations; and Medicine, which created doctors, who it appeared did not. (I didn't know then that most branches of medicine have an interventional aspect: cardiologists do cardiac catheterisation; gastroenterologists do endoscopies; respiratory doctors do bronchoscopies; and emergency medicine doctors and anaesthetists carry out intubations, among other procedures.) The idea of cutting into sleeping people was disturbing but I could already see it fitted medical school's focus on activities that were unacceptable in normal life: undressing people in public; moving things that hurt; touching dead bodies.

The basic principles of surgery were easier to understand than medicine. The surgeons drew diagrams. 'Excuse my terrible drawing,' they said. They added dotted lines to show where they planned to cut, or scribbled over bits they wanted to take away. Sometimes they drew on the patients, with a finger – 'We'll go in here, then we'll poke a tiny camera through here, there'll be three little holes – here, here and here.' As Berger says in *A Fortunate Man*, 'his tasks, however complex, are limited. They have a beginning and an end and can be checked. A technique, however fine, is always within known bounds.'

Surgery created wounds, openings which then needed to be 'closed', as the surgeons called it. At medical school, I was taught to suture on a square of pink latex. I practised for my exams on an orange (the students debated what provided the more lifelike experience, an orange or a banana; I found out when I had to stitch a human arm that it was neither). As a child, I was good at sewing: that is, I was good at making felt mice wearing bonnets. Suturing is not like sewing. The needle is often curved, and you hold it with a needle-holder, which looks like a pair of tweezers. Your other hand manipulates a pair of forceps. It was like eating a meal while holding your knife and fork with chopsticks. To tie a knot, you wrapped the suture around the needle-holder, looping it towards you, then away from you, then towards you. After a few loops, or 'throws', you got to say 'cut!', as on television.

Once the wounds were closed and dressed, and the anaesthetic had worn off, the surgeons sent their patients home, back into the community, where the practice nurses and the district nurses did wound care. They were the holders of the knowledge of what was normal and what was not. As the on-call GP, a message sometimes popped up on my screen: would you come and have a look at this wound? This meant not normal. I would go round to the nurse's room, fearing what I was going to see. I formed a biased view of wounds, as I only saw those that had gone wrong – infected, coming apart. I was careful about what I said, as the room was already full of distress and mistrust. By contrast, whenever anything healed we always commented on the quality and admired the stitches. 'Lovely and neat,' I said to Mr Smith as we looked at the scar on his abdomen. His expression was dubious. 'Will it get better than this?' he said. I said yes, because even if the scar didn't change, the patient's view of it usually did: he noticed it less, accepted it into his picture of himself, even if it was crooked.

Sometimes the surgeons inserted a drain, a temporary plastic tube to collect the fluid that can accumulate after an operation. The drain kept the wound dry and so helped it to heal. On first encounter, drains seemed bizarre. Where is all this liquid coming from? Why is it that colour? Is it meant to have bubbles in it? As a GP I saw drains less often as they were usually removed before the patient left hospital. But sometimes a patient was discharged with a drain still in place, for removal once the fluid had dried up, and it was clear that the patient hadn't always understood the surgeon's intentions. One day a daughter brought her mother in after the older woman's mastectomy. They were unhappy about the drain. The woman lifted her shirt to show me her chest, turning her face away as she did so. A tube stuck out of her skin where her breast had been, held in place with two thick sutures. The drain bottle rested in her lap, tucked inside a brightly patterned drawstring bag which was as unconvincing as all disguised medical equipment. I remembered a toddler on the ward who had refused the paediatric cannula dressings, his rage redirected at the smiling teddies printed on the plasters. 'No bear!' he would shout. 'No bear, no bear, no bear!'

'I want you to take it out,' said the daughter. 'She wants you to take it out, don't you?' she said to her mother. 'It's sucking the life out of her.'

At this time R was still training as a surgeon. He went to every operation he could. Some of the surgeons were odd, he said. One of the consultants rarely spoke until he started operating, and then he talked non-stop, but only to the organs. It's like they're his children, said R. 'Hello, Mr Spleen! Hello, Mr Pancreas! Oh, such a pretty gallbladder. Come out, darling, don't be shy.' One night, R assisted in a renal transplant. As soon as the surgeon joined the donor kidney to the recipient's blood vessels, it went pink, flushed with blood from its new circulation. 'And then it did a little pee!' said R. 'I *can* see why you might think the organs are alive. I mean, of course they're alive. Why you might think they're friends.'

One of the most senior surgeons struggled with life outside theatre; it was clear that the bowel made more sense to him than anything we said. He didn't like English food and chewed a cardamom pod instead of eating lunch. The pot-pourri smell combined with his accent and his moustache to make his patients suspicious. 'That foreign doctor,' an elderly lady said, 'foreign' meaning 'incompetent'. The patients made it plain they didn't understand what he was saying; they asked him to repeat himself. Often they would talk across him to the F1, so bypassing the specialist and directing their questions to the most ignorant person in the room. The consultant waited. Then he would lay his hand on his patient's abdomen (most doctors have to use a stethoscope to detect bowel sounds) and smile at the first piece of intelligible communication he'd had all day.

I strained to understand what was happening in theatre, even after reading most of a manual called *Assisting at Operations: A Practical Guide*, edited by a surgeon called Comus Whalan. 'Although it is only a small point, when you have a spare moment outside the operating theatre it is useful to check with a ruler that you know how long half a centimetre is. This seems to be one of those odd facts, which we often think we know, when we do not.' I was finding that there were a lot of these facts. 'Keep unnecessary movements of your hands and vocal cords to the minimum. In particular, do not play with the instruments.' 'Cut with the tips of the scissors ... if you cut with the mid-part of the blades, it is possible the tips may also inadvertently cut something else, perhaps the sort of something that should not be cut.' All I could think about was the sort of somethings that should not be cut.

Scrubbing made me nervous. The concept of sterile and non-sterile was so precisely mapped – the inside of the gown sterile but the outside not, this side of the table you could lean on but that side not. The operating department practitioners watched, and the meaner ones laughed. If you touched the wrong thing, they would sometimes shout at you. Any contamination and you had to take everything off – gown, gloves, mask – and start again. 'Put it all in the bin,' the ODP said. 'Wasted.'

I was a medical student when I attended my first operation. I came into the theatre to find the anaesthetist eating a KitKat. He had a copy of *The Times* folded open at the letters page, and was reading out a funny one to the ODP.

'I can't believe you can eat a KitKat in here,' I said.

'Thirty years of putting people to sleep, I could probably eat a three-course meal if there was anywhere to put the cutlery,' he said.

They were preparing for an arm operation. The patient, who had been slid from his hospital bed to the high operating table, put his hand up. He was worried they might have forgotten to knock him out, that someone might start cutting while he was still awake.

'We'll put you to sleep in a minute,' said the anaesthetist.

'All right, sir,' said the patient.

Minutes later, the anaesthetist put him to sleep. 'Count down from ten,' he said. As soon as he was out, the team covered him in drapes. The patient's grey hair poked out. The ODP attached a pleated tube, like a vacuum-cleaner hose, to a smaller green tube, which was then inserted into the patient's mouth. They laid a sheet of clear cellophane over his head; it rustled in the breeze from the fan. The room had its own microclimate, air conditioning, dry air, fans; none of it accidental. Theatres tend towards cold, hence the use of the Bair Hugger or 'forced air warming device', a kind of lilo pumped full of warm air. (Bair Hugger is the ubiquitous brand in British hospitals, despite the inventor having since come up with an alternative device called the HotDog. When I first heard the name I couldn't think what the theatre staff were talking about.)

Artificial ventilation doesn't look like normal breathing. The patient's chest heaves up and down in a mechanical way. At first it was difficult not to react to the learnt associations of a heaving chest – pain, distress. The students looked at the patient's head, checking to see if he was awake. The constant heavy movement startled us – it seemed like flinching.

Everything was draped except Mr Smith's arm. 'Can you pass me the scissors?' asked the surgeon.

'Do you want these, or a smaller pair?' said the scrub nurse. She was junior, training; her colleague stood behind her, advising. 'She'll want the smaller,' said the ODP.

The ODPs knew the size of every surgeon's hands. They knew what music each surgeon liked, and at what height she preferred her stool, and where to angle the light. The hierarchy is flatter now, but the senior member of the team's preferences are still accommodated in theatre, and the environment, chatty or hushed, will usually be set up to suit him or her, as will the music, which sometimes changed after the anaesthetic had taken effect – Magic FM to Wu-Tang Clan. 'No question I would speed, for cracks and weed,' crooned the orthopaedic registrar as he sponged iodine over an anaesthetised patient's hip. 'I have done my birth plan for the next one,' a friend told me after her caesarean. 'It's only got one item on it: no Ed Sheeran.' The ODPs tied the surgeons into their gowns, and replaced the gown with a clean one if there was any breach in the sterile field during the operation. I once watched an ODP jump forwards and catch a surgeon's scrub bottoms as they slid towards the floor (the pyjama knot had come undone). He reached round under the surgeon's gown, pulled his trousers back up to the right height and re-tied the knot. 'There you go, flower,' he said.

In the arm operation, the old man twitched. The surgeon waited, her knife just above the arm; a red line marked where she had started to cut. 'We have some responding,' she said. 'I'm running him very light,' said the anaesthetist. 'I'll give him some more, hold on.'

'You'd better look out,' the surgeon said to me. 'First operation I saw, and it was all that I wanted to do.'

A few months later, now attached to a colorectal team, I went to a bigger operation, a laparotomy. The patient was having part of his colon removed, or resected. The consultant had drawn us a sketch beforehand, with the familiar dotted lines to show the parts she intended to detach. Not long before this, a consultant had said to me, 'You are not a natural surgeon, I think.' This was a polite way of saying, you are an idiot. Before I went to the laparotomy, I thought that everything in the abdomen was going to be still, that the anaesthetic caused total paralysis. 'You thought it stopped your heart?' said one of the other students.

Now I could see the diaphragm rising and falling as the ventilator inflated and deflated the lungs. The bowels rose up into the wound like a pot about to boil over. Heat came out of the opening. Unlike those of the cold, faded cadaver, the tissues were hot and plump and brightly coloured. The registrar passed me a length of colon and asked me to hold it. As I picked it up, a ripple of peristalsis passed along the walls, the automatic muscle contraction that enables digestion. 'Wrongness,' my friend said when I told him this afterwards. 'Like you would pick up a snake?'

Out of theatre, the surgical trainees were distinguished by their shiny nails, from scrubbing, and their impulse to fiddle. It was still a job about using your hands, even as the robots were primed to take over. In one of my training jobs, I worked for an ENT team, doing everything except theatre; the before and after. I wrote up the notes in their doctors' office, which was as messy as usual. There was the same deflated lilo in the corner and the same half-eaten bag of Haribo on the windowsill for months. One day I came in to find lots of small new things: deformed paperclips, sculptural lumps of Blu-tack. 'It's Dr Smith's project,' the other F2 said. 'He's inventing a tool for getting foreign bodies out of ears. It's going to be revolutionary.' Dr Smith was keen to tell us about it. Getting soft things out of ears is easy: you can impale them on a tool called a wax hook and drag them out. But round items, like marbles, are harder. They spin when poked, and slip further out of reach. The ENT surgeons sometimes had to take children to theatre and give them a general anaesthetic in order to remove a bead. But what if, Dr Smith wondered, there was a tool with a flipper on the end, which could flick a foreign body out like the flipper in a pinball game? Or a tool with a sticky bit like the fishing game at the fairground?

Fiddling had given rise to some of the most useful inventions in medicine: things we used daily, without considering their ingenuity. 'If you were clever,' a surgeon said to me – we were standing next to an open abdomen and the surgeon was resting his hand on a length of colon, occasionally patting it – 'you'd have invented something by now. Like Fogarty. Guaranteed millionaire before he even qualified. Just from twiddling about with a bit of surgical glove.' (Thomas Fogarty, a scrub technician in Cincinnati in the 1940s, invented his eponymous arterial catheter by attaching the fingertip of a surgical glove to the end of a urinary catheter. When glue wouldn't stick, he used fly-fishing knots. Threading the catheter up the obstructed artery, inflating the balloon and then dragging it back out with the clot became a new procedure, balloon embolectomy, which revolutionised vascular surgery.)

We had recently moved to a new house, and soon after arriving I managed to snap the handle off the door of the shed. I asked a neighbour for help. He arrived with an ice axe and a monkey wrench. 'I use this at work,' he said, waving the wrench: he was an orthopaedic surgeon. We established that he didn't mean the actual tool he was holding, but rather something that looked like it. I stood about, waiting for him to bark 'AXE!' or 'WRENCH!' at me, but it took him two minutes to winkle the door open. 'I love operating,' he said.

As surgery involved kit, it also needed people to care for and understand kit; the specialty technicians. As a medical student I spent an afternoon at the fracture clinic, watching the plaster technicians work. One sewed stockinette into lengths. Another was cutting up adhesive felt to line a cast. The lead technician was mixing up different colours of plaster. I wondered if this was important. 'It's important for us: it gets boring without the colours. We've been doing some with glitter today,' she said.

She handed me a manual covered in splats of hardened plaster, *The Smith & Nephew Practical Guide to Casting*. It gave advice to anyone about to be incarcerated in a cast. 'Plan ahead!' suggested Smith and Nephew. 'Perhaps you should consider taking up a new hobby, like tapestry, or model making, or a new language.' The technician looked at the pictures with me. 'You won't see that much any more ... We hardly ever do that, very rare ... That's rare ...' she said, as I turned the pages. I came to a photograph of a baby with congenital hip deformities who had been bandaged up with his legs held apart. 'The frog!' she said. 'That's a nightmare for the mums, when they're nursing, can't fit him on your lap.'

This hospital differed from the technician's previous hospital. 'They did what you told them, at the last place. The thing about these patients is that they're *exceptionally* non-compliant. Let them out in plaster of Paris and they'll *destroy* it. Go roller-skating, go running, take it in the bath.'

'You have to explain everything in baby language,' she said. 'I had a patient with a fractured radius, common enough, got the plaster on, neat job, and she says, "Can I go on the sunbed with this?" and I'm like, "Why would you want to do that, you'll have a stripy arm, won't you?"'

Everything to do with equipment had its own craftspeople. They manipulated the standard form of each appliance to fit the unique shape and personality and habits of each patient. There were staff specialised in breathing equipment, orthotics, stomas, catheters, PEG tubes, artificial voiceboxes. The equipment was useless without the staff: no one else had their knowledge, their ability to translate the manufacturer's instructions into something that worked on an actual human. On my ENT job, I once spent an hour with the specialist nurse and the registrar, trying to mend an artificial voicebox. A spring-mounted part had flipped out, causing the valve to leak. It was like constructing a Kinder Egg model, coaxing one tiny piece to fit into another. As we poked at the part with an unfolded paperclip, the nurse told us that this was Mr Smith's second voice prosthesis, and that they'd just got it perfect for him when it had broken. 'When he loses his voice, he *really* loses his voice, if you see what I mean,' she said.

While surgery was focused on fixing and manipulating and physical kit, medicine preferred to solve puzzles with drugs. Pharmacology filled every student with dread, except the former pharmacist, now retraining as a doctor, who had the serenity of a man who'd already spent six years of his life phoning doctors to tell them they'd made a prescribing error.

Drugs quickly lost their romance. When I was a child, medicines were exciting. There were lots of medicines in stories. Children received spoonfuls of foul-tasting stuff that made them better. They bore it bravely. I mashed up leaves and petals in the garden to make tonics. This was real medicine, to me: retaining the potential for poisoning. Once my brother finished his years of fifteen pills with every meal, which we were not allowed to touch, we more or less forgot about his treatment. The medicine box at home still contained danger. A beige plastic cabinet with a red cross on the front, it hung high up on the bathroom wall. When the door opened a smell of Savlon came out. Only an adult could open it, but if I stood behind my mother I could glimpse inside. There was the brown plastic bottle of paracetamol with its child-proof click-click-click lid, and the spare capsules for the asthma inhalers, which underwent a controlled explosion inside the plastic device, releasing powder you could taste in your throat as it entered your windpipe, eaten and inhaled simultaneously, like a gastronomic experiment. A box of Elastoplast that lasted many years, as in our house you only got a sticking plaster if your leg fell off. Inside a plastic case that unscrewed into two parts was the thin glass thermometer with the silver line that only adults could see, that would poison you to death if you bit it. With the thermometer in my mouth I made my lips soft in case my jaw accidentally clamped. Once, the thermometer broke and a silver ball of mercury rolled across the floor. I wanted to play with it, but I didn't want to die.

Medical school introduced the standard encyclopaedia of drugs: the *British National Formulary*, or *BNF*, its tissue pages packed with miniature print, creating the immediate impression that there was not enough room for the information. Mode of action, indications, contraindications, side effects, complications. Twenty or more drugs in each class, with their generic names and their brand names, creating the paradox of the *BNF* – you cannot look up the drug you've forgotten unless you haven't forgotten it, as you need the name to find it. Even as we started pharmacology we knew we would never know it all. It was over before we'd begun.

You had to learn to pronounce the drugs. The patients couldn't, but they didn't care. The way they mispronounced told you how silly they found the word they were mangling. 'Bendroflumewhatsitcalled,' Mr Smith would tell you. But we were supposed to be infallible. You would see the panic flicker on a student's face when the registrar asked them to read out the drug chart. Bendroflumethiazide; amlodipine; omeprazole. There isn't an agreed way to pronounce a lot of medications. Down on the south coast, an F2 from a London medical school felt we were getting it wrong. 'In London we say "dyeCLOfenac". Not "DICKlofenac",' he explained. 'In Brighton we say "dickhead",' said the registrar. I was still coming to terms with drugs having both generic names and brand names (diclofenac gel is sold in chemists as Voltarol; it is also the analgesic ingredient in the arthritis drug Arthrotec).

The drug companies gave us things. Medical school was a time of gifts. Within a week of starting I owned a biro shaped like a bone with the word PFIZER printed on it. It was soon joined by a squeezy stress toy in the form of a kidney. They were giving us dog toys. We loved it. They also handed out Post-it notes, desk calendars and ID-badge holders. I noticed that the calendar missed off the national holidays ('About right,' the F2 said), and the pens didn't write very well. Still, free. Once a colleague produced a sachet of lubricating gel. 'Check this out!' he said. 'They're just giving them away in the lecture hall!' We ran. Doctors use lubricating gel for intimate examinations, or to facilitate interventions such as catheterisation. So what if there were tubes of KY brimming out of every drawer in the hospital? It wasn't the same.

The cornucopia increased when I started work. In my first job, we attended weekly grand rounds, a seminar held in the main lecture theatre. In the dark, with everyone's bleeps going off, grand rounds had an air of medical drama. In fact, it mostly consisted of PowerPoints about rashes, or scientific papers featuring many graphs. If you looked down the rows you could make out the motion of sixty-five pairs of jaws masticating free sandwiches. Food was the pharmaceutical companies' most powerful weapon. They no longer offered wine or restaurants, but rather a buffet of orange squash and Wagon Wheels, to be consumed while the drug rep took 'ten minutes of your time' to outline a breakthrough in diabetes treatment.

There was an obvious division between drugs that seemed to do something and drugs that appeared to do nothing. Adenosine, a medicine that hospital doctors give patients who are in new-onset or 'acute' heart block (that is, their hearts have suddenly started to miss a dangerous number of beats), is like an electric shock in a tablet: the patient may experience a sensation of impending death. This is a known side effect of the tablet and we were told to warn people about it. 'You may get a sensation of impending death. It's normal, and doesn't mean death is impending.' The medicine worked fast. The patient would look cartoonishly horror-stricken then immediately fine. The diuretic furosemide, given to remove fluid from the lungs in heart failure, also worked quickly when given intravenously, relieving the sensation of drowning as it was still running through. Salbutamol reversed the sensation of suffocation in minutes. All the anaesthetists' drugs did something obvious and usually alarming.

Other medicines were less obvious in their effects. Patients on beta-blockers were a reliable ward-round trick. The consultant would ask you to 'assess this patient's pulse'. You'd step forward, take the patient's wrist in your hand and look up at the clock. Within a few seconds you'd realise the pulse was improbably slow: could this be true, or were you counting wrong? Holding on, hoping for an answer to declare itself, the patient's wrist and your fingers would start to sweat. 'Are they bradycardic?' you'd try. 'Am I psychic?' the consultant would respond. This ritual would be followed by an attempt to recall the causes of a bradycardia – a pulse rate slower than sixty beats a minute – until someone remembered to look in the drug chart. 'Bisoprolol!' she shouted. 'Christ,' the consultant said.

Other drugs, especially the drugs we used in GP, appeared to do very little. The medicines we used to treat high blood pressure, heart disease and type 2 diabetes – blood pressure tablets, statins – were boring. Nor did it help that you couldn't see or feel the illness you were trying to prevent.

The drug companies did their best to confer personality. They made the tablets in different shapes and colours, and chose exotic names, like manufacturers trying to sell cars. But the experience of taking the medicine was still dull. Nothing happens when you take most pills – no palpable change in your health. If you feel a bit tired before you take 20mg of atorvastatin, you will feel a bit tired after it. You might go to the doctor occasionally and get a blood test – cholesterol, or HbA1C if you're a diabetic – but the whole experience is fundamentally abstract. It was unsurprising that patients got attached to particular brands, even if the active ingredients were identical. The taste or the colour of the tablet or the name on the box were all you had to differentiate this medicine from that. I was also a believer. For me, Beecham's Flu Plus, paracetamol formed into a fluorescent orange tablet, worked better than own-brand paracetamol, a dull white disc that powdered your fingers and lacked any bull's eyes or lightning bolts on the packet.

We arrived for our first-ever working day at the hospital ready to commit heroic acts of lifesaving. We carried stethoscopes and tourniquets. But the first nurse we saw did not ask us to restart anyone's heart. Instead, he handed us a pile of drug charts, each one labelled with a Post-it note 'REWRITE PLEASE :-)'.

Rewriting drug charts was tedious but essential. We had all been to lectures about drug errors, and been shown slides of charts where doctor handwriting had caused mistakes. But rewriting drug charts never happened in an environment conducive to concentration. It had to be done sitting down, which usually meant at the nurses' station, which meant sitting next to a phone. The phone would ring constantly. A sedentary doctor was a provocative sight in hospital. Soon more drug charts arrived, along with other administrative tasks. Now you were copying two charts at the same time, breaking occasionally to prescribe fluids for someone else. Every hospital liked things done in a different way, on a different style of chart, with the intravenous medications and antibiotics and insulin put in different places. Sometimes even in these olden times we prescribed on the computer, where a drop-down menu offered you fourteen different options for prescribing paracetamol and it was a minimum of five clicks per medicine – drug name, dose, frequency, route, indication.

Admission to hospital was a dangerous time. When patients came in, they needed their regular medications writing up, plus whatever else we were going to give them. It was often the middle of the night; the GP surgeries were closed. The patient could remember the colour of the pill they took, but not the name, or the dose. Or the carer handed you a plastic bag of medications; when you tipped them out in order to copy them onto a chart half had expired and the rest were in a bottle labelled with a piece of tape on which someone had written WATER PILLS. When I became a GP I realised that leaving hospital was also unsafe, as I received my patients' discharge letters. Now the medications were in a neat computerised list, but they no longer tallied with what the patient had been taking originally. Where had their warfarin gone? Stopped intentionally, or had someone forgotten to copy it down? Here was an antibiotic prescription labelled 'GP to continue'. Really? It wasn't just meant for the week they stayed in? How long were we meant to continue it for? Every discharge letter reminded me of being an F1, handed a stack of notes and told to 'do the discharges'. How could you know what had happened to this patient you might never have met? As an F1, I hadn't known what half the medications for chronic illnesses were even for: I'd never prescribed them. Blood pressure tablets, Parkinson's medicines, diabetes drugs – recurring names that meant little.

Drug allergies were problematic. 'Are you allergic to anything?' we asked every patient we met. ('Doctors!' said Mr Smith. I tried to make my laugh sound fresh.) People thought they couldn't have penicillin but couldn't remember why not. Sometimes they'd been told it had made them ill when they were infants. 'You'd have to ask my mother,' said an eighty-year-old. There is a distinction between an allergy and a predictable side effect – the former is potentially dangerous, the latter is not – but this distinction was hard to convey to a confused patient in the middle of the night.

One weekend, working as a medical F2, I went to see a ward patient who had become ill overnight. She had been admitted with dehydration after a bout of food poisoning. Now the nurses had bleeped for a doctor as she had a temperature of 40 degrees and rigors – uncontrollable shivering. When I got to her she looked unwell. She was drowsy and breathing fast; her skin was hot when I touched it. Listening to her chest, I could hear her heart beating at over a hundred beats a minute, and crackles at the bottom of her right lung as the airways popped open against the weight of secretions. I diagnosed pneumonia. I was pleased to have found something straightforward. I picked up the drug chart and prescribed an antibiotic called co-amoxiclav, to be given intravenously three times a day. I asked the nurse to give the first dose straight away.

I went across the corridor and into the cupboard that served as a doctors' office. I needed to request a chest X-ray for the patient, and I had to write an Hx/Ex/Imp and P in her notes. When I picked the notes up, an old drug chart fell out. **PENICILLIN ALLERGY** it said on the front. My heart rate doubled. 'She's allergic to penicillin!' I told the other on-call doctor. 'Bad,' he said. 'I saw a penicillin anaphylaxis once. Dead in ten minutes. Ugly.' My bleep went off. I was sure I was being bleeped back to a murder scene. I ran back to the ward and pulled the curtain open. The woman had her eyes closed; her drip arm was hanging over the side of the bed like David's painting of Marat lying dead in his bathtub. God almighty, I thought. I looked up at the drip stand; 0.9% Normal Saline, it said on the bag. The nurse came in. 'She's asleep. She's allergic to penicillin, so I didn't give it,' he said. 'I was bleeping you to tell you.'

General practice exposed my erroneous beliefs about how people took their medicines. Initially I proceeded as innocently as I had in hospital. I prescribed medicine to Mr Smith and assumed he took it. It didn't occur to me that I could be less than omnipotent. When Mr Smith returned, and his blood pressure, cholesterol and blood sugar were the same as they had been before, I increased the doses. Sometimes I changed the drug. I used an algorithm called the pain ladder to calibrate painkillers. Paracetamol not working, let us step up to codeine, and so on, until we reach morphine. There were other drug algorithms or ladders, for steroid creams and blood pressure drugs. A ladder was a welcome structure in the swamp of pharmaceuticals. It implied organisation. Management was always our medical goal. We didn't want to see reproachful labels in our patients' notes: 'poorly managed diabetes', 'poorly controlled hypertension'.

It was a while before I understood why many medications seemed to work better in hospital. It was because they were dispensed on a drug round, with a nurse giving Mr Smith his tablets more or less as prescribed, a beaker of water on the side. If you wrote or typed a medication on a chart you could generally assume it had entered the patient's body by a predictable route and at a predictable time. I had never needed to enquire further.

In the community, I soon learnt to ask. Tell me about your tablets, I said, trying to look like someone you'd want to confide in. 'Are you getting on OK with them? Any concerns?' Now, sometimes, I learnt how it was at home, rather than how I had chosen to believe it to be at home. Some obstacles were practical. Mr Smith couldn't get the pills out of the blister pack. The tablet disintegrated when he tried to score it in half. Some tablets were 'the size of a horse pill' and got stuck when he tried to swallow them. Others were tiny and slipped out of his fingers and fell down the sink or got lost in the rug. Pills were literally bitter; suspensions invariably tasted disgusting. It was difficult to take the medication at the same time every day, as Mr Smith worked shifts. 'Take one tablet each morning half an hour before food' sounded easy, but Mr Smith already woke at five to leave for work and now we were asking him to wake at four-thirty instead, an additional thirty dark minutes in which to reflect on the tediousness of medication. Some patients didn't like or felt they couldn't afford the prescription charge (£9.35 per item per month for adults under sixty, free if you qualified for an exemption certificate). They let me know that they thought they shouldn't have to pay, or that they'd paid already, as didn't they pay taxes?

Then there were more nebulous interferences, the patient's beliefs about the medicine they were meant to be taking, which our training had liked to call ideas, concerns and expectations. 'Did you get the ICE?' the trainer would ask at the end of a consultation while I suppressed my own ICE about the grammar of contemporary general practice. 'You're going to do GP?' one of the surgical trainees once said to me, 'With all that ICE stuff? I could *never*. I think you have to be a particular type of person.' She looked at me with her head tilted sympathetically, the way a GP might. 'No doubt,' I said.

Sometimes you knew what people believed about a particular medicine. Their beliefs were usually somewhat true, sometimes, or for some people, or on some occasions. Statins made your muscles ache, blood pressure tablets made you dizzy, laxatives caused diarrhoea, anti-depressants ensnared you in dependency, simple analgesia 'doesn't work' but stronger analgesia would lead to buying heroin on the street. Some medicines had such an infamous reputation that it was hard to get patients to take them (while another group of patients could not be persuaded off them). Many patients knew opioids to be lethal and addictive – which they were, when used wrongly. Sometimes, fearing overdose, dying patients reduced the prescribed doses of oral morphine to half and so had half-treated pain. On home visits I carried an empty syringe in my bag so I could use it to demonstrate how much Oramorph to take. Fill up a whole syringe, and then another whole syringe, it's fine to drink both, no it's not dangerous. 'Quite safe!' I said, just stopping myself from squirting the pretend medicine into my mouth.

There was a widespread dislike of taking any medicine at all. Medicine was felt to be bad for you. Along with this came a belief that, regardless of their individual effects or indications, too many different tablets could be harmful. Each person's 'too many' differed, but if Mr Smith felt he had been prescribed an excessive number of medications, he might elide a few, scaling himself back down to whichever number he felt to be safest *for him*.

Our poor explanations made everything worse. We mentioned side effects without contextualising their relative frequency or rarity, so that for a while everyone I started on amlodipine said their ankles were swollen (in trials this happened to about two per cent of patients. I began saying that amlodipine could *very occasionally* cause ankle swelling.) Or we forgot to mention side effects altogether, so the patient stopped taking their antibiotics, fearing their loose stools meant harm. We didn't tell Ms Smith that her periods might stop while she was on the pill but that they would restart afterwards, her fertility unimpaired. 'It is worth telling everyone,' said my GP trainer, 'that the blood does not *build up inside*.'

We forgot to explain that medication would be lifelong, and so Mr Smith took his blood pressure pills until the prescription ran out and didn't collect any more. 'I completed the course!' he said when I saw him. He sounded annoyed. 'I didn't realise you wanted me to go on and on and on with it.' Or he stopped as soon as he got an improved blood pressure reading, rationally concluding that the medicine had worked. Telling people to read the leaflet inside the packet was not enough. Everyone read the paragraph about rare side effects but skipped the administration instructions. Ms Smith came in because she felt bloated. She wondered if it was a side effect of her pill. She had switched from the combined contraceptive pill (two hormones per tablet, taken daily, with a seven-day break per month) to a different type of contraceptive pill called the mini-pill (one hormone, taken daily, no breaks). She had omitted the new tablet for a week each month, as this was what she had always done. We had referred to both drugs as 'the pill'. Missing seven mini-pills each month puts you at risk of pregnancy. She was pregnant.

Changing the administration route of familiar drugs was risky. My colleague tried to overcome Miss Smith's fear of morphine by prescribing opioid patches instead. He forgot to emphasise the taking off and sticking back on part of the process. When I visited Miss Smith she said her pain was much better. When I asked to see her patch, she rolled up her sleeve. She had a week's supply of buprenorphine stuck in a row down her arm. It reminded me of an afternoon, years previously, in hospital. I had sent a medical student to take blood from a patient. When he didn't come back, I went to see if he was OK. I found him labelling bottles next to the patient's bed. There were wrappers all over the floor, and the patient had four plasters on her arm: one for each of the laboratory test samples. I went back to apologise after I'd taken the student away. 'I tried to tell him you can just take one syringe of blood and divide it into different bottles, but he didn't believe me,' the patient said.

A few months after the buprenorphine patch-up, a couple came in together for an appointment. One night, while they were asleep in bed, her HRT patch had detached itself. It had restuck itself to her husband's back, where it remained unnoticed for a week. They were concerned about his masculinity, 'going forward'.

On home visits, when I asked patients to show me where they kept their medicine, I found evidence of how much medicine patients were not taking. There were boxes of laxative stacked in a cube on top of the fridge. Packets of calcium supplements fell out of the cupboards. In every nursing home there would be at least one resident with semi-dissolved calcium supplements coating their tongue. If you'd brought a student on the visit you could ask them what they thought the white exudate was and wait for them to diagnose thrush. (I knew this was babyish. It went along with 'Why have this patient's thighs turned blue?', to which the answer was dye transference from denim rather than dermatomyositis, and then you got to say the saying about hoof prints.)

There were mix-ups even when patients took their medicines as prescribed. People over-ordered through fear of running out, or in deference to lifelong hoarding instincts. Others were the victims of pharmacist or doctor malfunction. Mrs Smith asked me to remove the paracetamol from her repeat prescription. 'I can't stop the chemist sending it. I've got enough at home to suicide the whole estate,' she said. The chemist couldn't accept it back, she told me. If you bring it in, we can get rid of it for you, I said. 'That's all right,' she said. 'My son has to pay for his, so I'm supplying him. I said: "Knock on my door, I'll do you a deal."' She looked at me. 'I'm not *really* charging him.'

Prescribing medication as a GP could be demoralising. 'You're trying to poison him,' said a patient's wife, before I'd even formed the words 'Any concerns?' 'Not you *personally*,' she said. I envied the supplement industry. No one seemed suspicious of their treatments: on the contrary, they paid to have more of them. There were no qualms about polypharmacy either. The more supplements you took, the healthier you would become. No one seemed aggrieved when CoEnzyme Q10 failed to remedy their exhaustion.

I tried to reassure people. I mentioned evidence, research. 'This has all been tested,' I said. 'I wouldn't be suggesting this if I didn't feel it might be useful.' I stressed my disinterest. 'It is not down to me to tell you what to do with your health,' I said, explicitly contradicting centuries of doctors before me. I stopped mentioning testing when I realised the idea made people uncomfortable. I remembered a video I'd watched at medical school. A doctor in a mad-professor outfit – white coat buttoned askew – bent over a baby in a crib. He took out what looked like a cartoon hatpin and poked the baby's foot. The baby jerked his foot back (a normal reflex) and began to wail. The professor picked him up and put him over the shoulder of his white coat. *There, there, sweet baby*, he said. As the screen cut to a picture of Bowlby's monkeys clinging to their sticks, a voice-over explained that the baby was developmentally normal. 'Those experiments would not be ethical now,' the lecturer said, turning the video off. 'So much of what we did would not be ethical now.'

Just occasionally there was an issue with over-compliance. There is a category of bone protection medicines called bisphosphonates which can damage the oesophagus if they reflux back out of the stomach. For this reason, bisphosphonates come with the instruction to remain upright for half an hour after ingestion. Sitting upright in bed is good enough, I said to Mrs Smith, after her husband told me she was spending an hour a week standing completely still in the middle of the sitting room, willing the tablet to digest. 'She looks like a heron,' he said. 'You said it could burn a hole,' she said to me. 'I didn't want to burn a hole, so I did exactly what you said.'

Women and Babies

The GP trainees acknowledged that obstetrics and gynaecology was useful for training, but we also knew it to be busy. This meant we were pleased if we were allocated the post, but also wished we had been given something quieter. Hospital gynaecology takes care of all aspects of women's health: dysfunctional bleeding, urinary incontinence, cancer, infertility. I hadn't realised that it also dealt with problems in early pregnancy – at this hospital, any problem occurring before twenty weeks' gestation.

As a medical student I had encountered an early-pregnancy problem only once. It was during an afternoon in A&E. A nurse had sent me to find a drip stand. Walking past the bays, I saw a man's head sticking out from one of the curtains, trying to get someone's attention. It reminded me of waitressing, the way people tried to catch your eye, and you knew they were doing it but could pretend not to have seen. I avoided his eye, although I wouldn't have acknowledged this to myself. Perhaps I thought I was busy. Eventually I stopped. Can I help? I said, knowing that it was unlikely that I could. He brought me behind the curtain. A woman was lying on her side on a trolley, holding her knees to her chest. 'She's thirteen weeks. She was thirteen weeks. It's a lot of blood, she's leaking,' he said. 'Have you got something?' There was no chair in the cubicle. He crouched at the end of the trolley and put his head on the woman's feet. I'm so sorry, I said. I went to find a towel or a sheet. You need an IncoPad, said a CSW when I asked her. I added the word to my hospital vocabulary, which I was hoping would one day allow me to pass as a doctor. There were no spare chairs.

One in four pregnancies end in miscarriage, the registrar told us on our first day as GP trainees in gynae. This ward was for that intense subsection of gynaecology that dealt only with pregnancies: miscarriages, morning sickness, ectopics and terminations. Within weeks of starting the job, pregnancy had come to seem fraught. I knew this was observational bias: all I saw was trouble, therefore pregnancy itself must be troublesome. I could usually manage this hospital distortion of normality – I knew most lumps were not cancer and most coughs were not TB. Until I became pregnant myself, and the biased version of events was all I could think about. Each week the NHS sent me a cheery email updating me on the fetus's progress – now it was the size of a pea, now the size of a walnut, now it could wave a tiny hand – and each week my brain worked through a parallel list instead. Ectopic pregnancy, molar pregnancy, inevitable miscarriage, fatal fetal anomaly.

Gynaecology clerking followed a familiar routine. First you took a history. This was also when you met the patient's partner, or friend, or aunt. It was essential to ask who the other person was, or you would call the girlfriend the mother or the brother the boyfriend. 'I'm her grandfather,' a man said to me. 'I know it seems weird. I'm like her dad, though. Which also sounds weird.' Then you carried out an examination. The women often spoke about 'down below', though sometimes they used the mad words for vagina – 'tuppence', 'foof', 'lady bits'. Often the patient said, This is embarrassing, and I would explain that I was not embarrassed, which was true. My list of embarrassments had changed. They now included any situation in which I might be revealed as incompetent to a spectator; unfamiliar clinical problems that would oblige me to guess a response; and having to phone a consultant about any topic. In practical terms I no longer distinguished between a vagina and an ear – they were both hard to see into.

To perform a VE, or a vaginal examination, you needed to be able to use a speculum, a plastic tool that props the vagina open so you can see the cervix, which medicine confusingly translated as 'the neck of the womb'. (I had been a GP for three years when I realised, while talking with a patient, that some women thought their vaginal canal was the neck of the womb. Which does make sense.) I didn't really learn to use a speculum until the start of my gynaecology rotation. Prior to that I basically learnt to mime with it. I would explain what I was going to do, gain consent, slide the speculum into the patient's vagina, see a blur of pink flesh, and say, 'All seems well.' Starting my gynae job didn't render me magically competent. The walls of the vagina still bowed in on each other, collapsing the view. Even if you could see to the end, the cervix rarely looked like the doughnut featured in textbooks, and it was often elusive. It hung down or rose up and sometimes appeared to be leaning sideways. 'It'll pop into view,' the gynae nurse said, coaching me as she chaperoned. She suggested manoeuvres as I nudged the speculum back and forth. 'Have her put her fists under her bottom,' she said. 'Get her to do a little cough.' She smiled up at the patient. 'Just pretend you're at the worst yoga class ever.'

The transition to competence occurred invisibly, as it had with every other clinical skill. I never saw a cervix, I was never going to see a cervix, and then suddenly I saw the cervix every time I looked for one. 'As plain as the nose on your face,' said the nurse when I shared the miracle. 'It also feels like your nose, interestingly,' she said.

It was fortunate my skills had improved, as gynae required a lot of vaginal examinations. If a woman was pregnant and bleeding, we usually examined the cervix, which we hoped would be closed. If it was open, an inevitable miscarriage was taking place. Sometimes tissue got stuck in the cervical opening, the 'os'. This stimulated the vagal nerve and caused a phenomenon called cervical shock, in which the patient suddenly became very unwell. I had learnt about cervical shock at medical school. As the lecturer scrolled through her slides, my neighbour drew cartoons of the different kinds of shock in his notebook – septic, haemorrhagic, hypovolaemic. The shocked cervix was a doughnut in tears. But I didn't believe it was a real thing until my first week of gynae.

The nurses asked me to clerk a woman who had been admitted to the ward with bleeding in her second month of pregnancy. The woman was giving me an account of events when she stopped and said she felt ill. 'God, that hurts!' she said. Her face went white. 'Christ,' said her partner, leaning over her. I felt her pulse. It seemed to be less than fifty beats a minute. The CSW took her blood pressure – 90/60. Was the patient haemorrhaging? I lifted up the blanket fearfully but the sheets were still white. How could she have low blood pressure *and* a low heart rate – why hadn't the heart speeded up to compensate? 'Please can you get the nurse, and tell her it's urgent?' I said to the CSW. One of the gynae nurses came immediately – I sometimes thought they stood outside the doors, protecting their patients from the new batch of doctors. You need to do a VE, she said, tipping the bed so that the patient's head was down. 'A vaginal exam?' I said, trying to convey that I was lost. The nurse explained to the patient in a way that I would also understand what to do. 'The doctor's just going to check the neck of the womb for you, and make sure it's clear,' she said. 'Sometimes tissue and blood can get stuck there and make you feel very ill.' She handed me a speculum and talked to the patient. 'OK, feet together, darling, drop your knees out to the sides for me, are you OK for the doctor to do this, she's just going to pop it in now, that's it, I'm just handing her some little forceps, you won't feel them, OK, this might cramp a little as she clears the obstruction, *there*, now you feel better, don't you?' I put some red tissue into the cardboard bowl the CSW was holding out and looked at the woman. She had transformed back into a regular patient, rosy and alert. 'What the fuck happened there?' her partner said. He looked faint.

The language on gynae was gross. 'She's had a vag hysterectomy,' said one of the nurses, handing over. 'Please don't say "vag",' I said. I felt even primmer than I sounded. 'Grim, isn't it?' she said. 'I hate the word "discharge".' The nurses started to list words that made them squeamish. 'Lubrication!' said one. 'Hygiene products!' 'God, remember Dr Smith?' one of them asked. Dr Smith was not a native English speaker. During a routine consultation he had asked a patient to take off her panties so he could examine her. The nurse who had been chaperoning came out sparkling. 'Who the fuck says *panties*?' she said. 'Ever after, we would bleep him: "Is Doctor Panty there, please? I have a lingerie enquiry for him."'

The medical language sounded dated. Some doctors still used the old terminology, calling miscarriage 'spontaneous abortion'. The miscarried fetus was 'the products of conception', or just 'the products'. This was how we wrote in the notes, not how we spoke to the patients. For the patient, the fetus was almost always a baby (although not always. 'Please just take it away,' said a fifteen-year-old who had come for a termination.)

We looked after terminations and miscarriages on the same

ward. 'Please be very mindful which room you are in,' the nurses said on the first day. I checked the patient's identity before knocking on the door and again on entering and sometimes I had begun the history when I found I wanted to check a third time. Recognising that this was madness did not stop the urge. 'Yay! More opportunities for *horrific* error!' said the GP registrar who had started with me.

One morning I was pushing my daughter to nursery when the wheels of the buggy raised a cloud of flies. There was a dead baby bird on the pavement. It was featherless, rolled up like a cigar, with the goggle eyes of a fetus. 'Why is it sleeping?' my daughter asked. 'It's not asleep, it's dead,' I said. She was pleased with this. 'It's dead, it's dead!' she sang.

At work later that morning, I clerked a patient and went to the nurses' station to write up the notes. There was a specimen bottle on the desk in front of me. 'Products,' said the nurse. I picked up the bottle and wiggled it, trying to see what was in it. The tiny red blob inside became a shape. Two upper limbs lifted out like wings and two spindly legs flapped like a tadpole's. I saw fetuses all the time on Facebook, we all did now, fuzzy ultrasound images posted with captions: 'Waving hello!', 'Thumbs up!' This fetus would never become a person, unlike the images on the internet. I was transfixed. 'She wants a funeral,' said the nurse, watching me looking at the bottle. 'Little thumbprint, it'll only need a matchbox.'

Hospital gynaecology was a surgical specialty, and so along with our ward work the juniors were often called to assist in theatre. The 'assisting' was not skilled: it consisted of holding some things still and other things out of the way. You had to do it even if your career choice involved never setting foot in a theatre again.

The first gynae operation I assisted at was a laparoscopic salpingectomy. The patient's fertilised egg had failed to waft along to the uterus, but instead had implanted into her fallopian tube, causing an ectopic pregnancy. As with all ectopics, there was a danger it would rupture; the resulting bleeding can kill the patient very quickly. An ectopic pregnancy was always urgent. If the patient showed any signs of worsening – falling blood pressure, rising heart rate, increasing pain – it became an emergency. Ms Smith had been admitted at around eleven in the evening, and the gynaecologists soon decided she needed surgery. The plan now, at one in the morning, was to remove her fallopian tube through small cuts in her abdomen. My job was to sit on a stool between the unconscious patient's legs and keep the uterus at the correct angle by exerting pressure on a pair of forceps that the consultant had clipped to Ms Smith's cervix. In front of me I could see the underside of the surgeons' chins. The monitor showing the operation was directly above my head; I could just see it if I swivelled until my neck popped. In the West End my seat would have been classified as RESTRICTED VIEW, one with a pillar in front of it, or an aerial view of the actors' hair. Soon the operating department practitioner turned the lights down, to allow the surgeons to see the monitor better, and when the darkness fell all the theatre staff stopped talking.

The registrar made a nick in the patient's tummy button and pushed a trocar through the hole. 'Gas, please,' she said. Inflating the abdomen with carbon dioxide separates the organs from one another to give the surgeon room to manoeuvre (ordinarily the abdominal contents are squashed in tightly: insufflation works like inflating a bouncy castle, pushing everything apart).

The screen went white as the registrar examined her gloved hand with the camera, checking the focus. Then there was a flash of the consultant's face as the camera waved past him, on its way in. I looked back up the table. The consultant was finicking over one of the incisions; the registrar was holding her tools still, waiting for him. 'OK, go now, go now!' he said. The light of the laparoscope spread a glow like a scuba diver's torch and lit up a cave. Under the inflated dome of the abdominal wall the fallopian tube was bulging like a sea anemone. 'Intact,' said the registrar, meaning that the ectopic hadn't ruptured. 'Good.' She bagged it up and winched it up and out and put it in a kidney dish.

Once they'd passed twenty weeks' gestation, pregnant women moved into the realm of the obstetricians. Their problems changed from ectopics and miscarriage to premature labour and pre-eclampsia. As obs and gynae juniors, we covered both disciplines and tried to keep the distinctions clear in our heads.

As a medical student, obstetrics was mainly frustrating. To pass the course, we had to 'deliver' a certain number of babies, which meant being in the room when the baby came out. The students waited in the midwives' office on the labour ward; there were not enough chairs, so we sat on the floor. A whiteboard on the wall listed the names of the women who were currently in labour. Next to each name was a box in which the midwives wrote in obstetric code. Each woman was a Gx Px, with G being gravidity – the number of pregnancies the woman had ever had, and P being parity – the number of pregnancies she had delivered after the threshold of viability (in the UK, twenty-four weeks). A midwife explained the terminology. 'What am I?' he asked us. 'Correct. I am G0 P0. As I am a man. But never assume,' he said. The board was dense with acronyms: ARM – artificial rupture of membranes; SROM – spontaneous rupture of membranes; VBAC – vaginal birth after caesarean. The progress of labour was expressed in cervical dilatation. 14:50 3cm; 16:00 6cm. We willed our allocated patients to progress, to hurry to delivery so we could attend and get our logbooks ticked. You couldn't leave the labour ward for even a moment, as if you did you could guarantee that your square would flick to SVD or LCSC – meaning the woman had just had her vaginal delivery or a caesarean section *without you*, and now you had to start all over again.

On a summer day, my allocated patient, a teenager, G1 P0, a 'nullip' as the midwives called the first-timers, was midway through labour. The midwife had sent me to sit in her room for a while as she was screaming. 'See if you can calm her down,' said the midwife. I doubted I could. I had the sketchiest sense of what normal labour was, and even in its normal aspects it seemed something to scream about. I arrived at the same time as the teenager's friend, who was holding a cardboard cupholder. 'It'll be OK, hon. Seriously, you need to chill,' said the friend. 'Ah, Macky Ds,' sighed the midwife. The teenager was frightened of needles and frightened of examinations; even touching her arm made her scream. She shuddered and cried during the epidural then started screaming 'take it out!' when the registrar inserted a speculum so that she could sample some blood from the baby's scalp. The blood sample showed the baby was distressed. The registrar told the patient she needed a c-section.

We wheeled the teenager to theatre. Her boyfriend walked next to the trolley with his head down. We could all hear the girl's teeth chattering. In theatre, she continued to shiver and plead. 'It's all right, sweetheart, it'll be all right,' said the anaesthetist. 'I'm just going to put this here, darling, you won't feel any pain I promise, no pain,' said the other anaesthetist. All the staff darlinged her, but she couldn't be comforted. She had lost her voice from screaming so much, and now when she screamed only a husking noise came out. Her feet rubbed together as though they had taken on the job of handwringing. The friend talked to the boyfriend. 'Just look away when they start – turn your head, you don't have to look, it's OK.' The boyfriend looked white. They got the drape on, with the hole centred on the girl's abdomen, and the corners clipped up to make a screen. The midwife came to the girl's head, took her hand and stroked her arm. 'Now come on, lovey. Enough now. It's about your baby. It's important.' The registrar, a Syrian woman in an operating headscarf, started sponging the girl's stomach with brown disinfectant, and then took a knife and cut through the first layer of skin and fat. The girl made her husk noise, her mouth open like a cat.

We looked at the registrar and back at the girl. Is this normal? Should she be crying out? Procedures often felt like this: no one free to explain anything, and no opportunity to ask. When was it ever appropriate, in front of a patient, to say 'Are you sure that's normal?' or 'Isn't the baby a funny colour?' or 'Were you expecting so much blood?' We looked at everyone's faces, to see if they looked worried. The girl was writhing – as much as she could writhe, tethered by the blood pressure cuff and partially paralysed by the spinal anaesthetic. 'No! Pain! There's pain!' she said. Which fitted with the wound opening in the lower end of her stomach. 'There's no pain, sweetheart. I told you you'd feel it, but that's *pressure*,' said the anaesthetist to the girl. He made faces to his colleague, who nodded, yes, it's working, she can't feel anything. The obstetrician made another cut. 'No! No! No!' strangled the girl. 'OK, wait,' said the anaesthetist. 'Listen, darling, seriously: can you feel *pain* or can you feel *pressure*? I know it feels strange, but is it *pain* you're feeling?' 'No! No! No!' said the girl.

A minute later, the anaesthetist said 'GA', and the boyfriend and the friend were ushered out, and the girl was asleep. Three minutes after that, the registrar was pulling the sides of the wound apart – in a caesarean, you tear the tissues with your hands, which looks brutal but allows better healing as the ragged edges knit back together more readily than the smooth edges of an incision. The registrar put her hands in and pulled. The head was born. She kept pulling, and out slithered the baby. The registrar cut the cord. She handed the baby to the midwife, who took it to an incubator in the corner and scrubbed at it with a towel for five seconds, then sucked at its mouth with a suction device, then took its head in her hands and clamped an oxygen mask over its mouth, all the time scrubbing, while the baby tipped one way and another. Finally, it made a mewling sound. It had none of the bounce of the new-borns I'd seen before. But the midwife was happy. 'Who wants a cuddle?' she said.

I put out my arms. The towel was wrapped tightly round the baby, leaving a porthole for her face, which looked like a face pressed against glass – flattened, mouth slack. I thought she wasn't breathing, but then saw the edges of her nostrils moving. 'She's just full of Mum's anaesthetic, sleepy girl,' said the midwife, looking over. The registrar had finished suturing and the ODPs were tidying up, pulling off the drapes and clattering equipment into the bins. The patient whom everyone was now calling Mum was still asleep. I held the baby and waited to find out what to do with her next.

That summer I went to Sri Lanka and spent time on elective in a rural hospital there. 'Birth is the same everywhere, what do you want to see for?' said the obs and gynae SHO as I followed him to the labour ward. He was wearing a plum-coloured shirt with a fresh sweat patch under each arm. The labour ward had a concrete floor and concrete walls with squares cut for windows, which were not glazed. On a table by the window, on a heat mat which seemed hot enough to cook on, lay a newborn baby, brown with blood. He smelt of iron and antiseptic, and his head was tubular at the crown from a suction delivery. On the bed behind us, his mother was being sutured, her legs hanging apart. The consultant was peering at the woman's perineum. A nurse stood next to the bed, holding a stick with a bloody swab on the end of it. She smiled at us when we came in. The woman rolled her head to look at us; her cheeks were swollen from crying. I stood next to the heat mat with the paediatricians as they chatted, in Sinhala with English medical words – umbilicus, ventouse, twenty-four-hour observation. There was blood dripping from the end of the bed. Through the window, the bougainvillea in the hospital yard looked dusty. Two women walked their babies about. A row of surgical gloves dried on the fence.

The next day, we did a ward round. The women lay on their beds in a row. The last bed had a curtain drawn around it. Outside the curtain there was a table with a washing-up bowl on it. In the bowl was a crumpled piece of checked cloth, one of the cloths that the women brought with them to use as coverlets, and towels, and bags for carrying belongings and babies. The consultant leant over and flicked the cloth open. A grey face appeared. The baby was frowning, and its mouth was pursed. I didn't understand why the baby had its face covered until the consultant put the cloth back, and I realised it was dead. I asked when it had been born. The mother had been induced after developing high blood pressure; the baby had been stillborn that morning. It was thirty-two weeks' gestation and weighed one and a half kilograms. The consultant explained that this wasn't that small. 'As long as they're above one kay-gee, they'll usually do all right. Some of these maids are thirty-six kilos – they're as small as children, right? You aren't going to get a big baby out of a tiny mother like that. Very poor nutritional status, very poor.'

On the labour ward there was a row of four beds, and in one of these a woman was labouring. Her black hair had been rubbed out of its plait by the movement of her head on the pillow and was in a haze around her face. Her flowered maternity dress was pushed up to her armpits. Three nurse orderlies stood beside her. Every two minutes, her sobbing built up to a cry, she took hold of a foot in each hand, and pushed until her face grew congested. The chief orderly spoke to her in Sinhala.

The woman's perineum was a sheet with an aperture through which there was an occasional glimpse of the baby's dark hair. The baby was not coming out. One orderly put her gloved hand in and wiped it around the baby's head. Another pressed on the woman's stomach. The woman scuffed her head on the pillow until her hair crackled. The orderlies chatted to each other. The SHO asked me where I was studying and frowned when I told her: 'I haven't heard of a medical school in that place.'

The orderlies were watching the clock. After half an hour, one pressed a plastic trumpet to the labouring woman's stomach to listen to the baby's heart. The house officer was watching the clock too; she spoke through to the next-door ward, ending in English, 'Half-hour well past now, just to warn you guys.' The SHO came in. He washed his hands and pulled on a single surgical glove, and leant over the woman. His phone rang. He took it out of his pocket with his ungloved hand, said something into it and threw it on the bed behind him. The nurse draped a cloth over the patient's lifted knee so he could lean on her without messing his clothes. His tie dangled over her stomach. He pushed his gloved hand into the woman and made the same unscrewing gesture as the orderly, but more forcefully, as if trying to get the lid off a jar. Water and blood fell out on to the bed, and the patient's face scrunched up. Then he pushed down on her stomach with both hands. The bed rocked on the floor. The orderly made an episiotomy cut and a second after that the baby shot out, a long bluish-white object, its face covered in the caul. It looked like an insect in a chrysalis. The orderly snatched it up and sawed through the cord with scissors and ran with the baby to the heat mat by the window. The woman on the bed lay with a hand sticking out over each side of the mattress and cloths heaped between her legs.

The orderly scrubbed at the baby with a cloth and the doctor poked its nose and mouth with a noisy suction tube. The baby gulped. Then it cried, and at once, like blowing into a balloon, it was taut all over, kicking its feet, thrashing its hands, struggling to get out of the oxygen mask the house officer was holding over its nose. Everyone laughed. Four thousand babies were born at this hospital each year – more than three hundred a month.

My obstetrics and gynae post happened to be my first job after coming back from my own maternity leave, and the job was in the hospital in which my son had been born. I had come in thirteen days after my due date, to be induced. A midwife showed me into a room and then she went away for several hours. At last she came back and put in a pessary to start off labour. She took me to a different room with a hospital bed. It was like going into any patient's room, except there was no patient in the bed, as I was the patient. I felt unsure about getting into the bed, as this was not something I would ever do at work. I didn't know what to do with myself, not being ill. R left. Nothing happened. I googled SIGNS OF IMPENDING LABOUR on my phone. Eventually, at midnight, I went to sleep. I woke up with cramps at 3 a.m. It was painful but not unbearable. It seemed most comfortable to kneel on the floor next to the bed with my head on the mattress. I got a paper towel from the dispenser by the sink and made a mark for each contraction. The pen marks warped on the bumpy paper. I don't know what I was counting for; perhaps I was just used to making lists in hospitals. At 5 a.m., I pressed the bell and explained I had pain. I didn't feel confident diagnosing contractions. The midwife came back with two paracetamol and a cup of water. I waited for the day to start, for company and for a plan. In hospital there is always a P:, if you wait long enough.

It turned out that labour did not obey this rule. There was a plan, but it was constantly revised. Doctors came in and had conversations with the midwife, who sat at the end of my bed. The midwife went away and came back. The ward round came in, and I watched the F1 writing in the notes and guessed the two young doctors carrying rucksacks were actually medical students. At lunchtime I qualified for the labour ward, so we moved rooms again. A porter came with a wheelchair for me. The midwife and R walked behind us. We filled the lift immediately, and the door closed. 'Not long, we'll be there in a minute!' said the midwife as we waited to move. The doors slid open to reveal a man holding a car-seat and a woman holding a baby. 'No, sorry!' the midwife said to them, pressing the button again.

In the new room, things went downhill. Suddenly the midwife pressed the emergency buzzer: the baby's heart rate had dropped. Lots of people ran in. After looking at the CTG trace, everyone left again. The heart rate had gone back to normal. The consultant came to discuss 'options'. A caesarean was becoming likely, but she thought it a bad idea. 'Think of your future obstetric career,' she said. I was confused: I wasn't planning to be an obstetrician. 'I mean the babies after this one – every time you have a caesarean, the risks go up.' It was hard to think of babies to come while the current baby was not being born. Ten minutes later, the midwife pressed the buzzer again, and everyone came back. This time there was shouting. 'I told you we should have had her in before!' the midwife said. 'This is ridiculous!' They unplugged the bed, and we were on a high-speed trolley chase to theatre, with the registrar reading a consent form at my head.

I could only remember bits of H's birth. I remembered the ceiling lights flying past like pylons as we went down the corridors, and worrying that the trolley was going to break the doors as we bust them open, and thinking someone had taken a photo when the anaesthetist's diamond ring flashed in the operating theatre lights. I could remember the cold spray icing my skin, and the anaesthetist saying 'Here? Here? How about here?' as she sprayed it on my torso to establish the anaesthetic level. I couldn't remember the baby being born. On the other side of the room, I saw his head jiggling as they rubbed him with a towel. They brought him over and put him next to my head, but I didn't feel I was the safest person to hold him, as they had just had to remove him from the unsafe environment of myself, and also I was having an operation, and I did not think you were supposed to hold babies during operations.

As with every new medical job, I was in unhappy anticipation for a long time before I started obs and gynae, although this time was worse, as maternity leave meant I had been out of any workplace for months. I began on nights, which increased my worry. The baby is up all night anyway, I reasoned with myself. On my first day back, I took H to nursery in the morning, then went home and tried to sleep. I couldn't sleep. I picked H up at five and gave him his tea. R came home at six-thirty. I put on a skirt and a shirt, my work clothes, and drove to the hospital; my shift started at eight. I drove around the blocks surrounding the hospital until I found a parking space. I put a pound in the meter and bought a ticket to cover me for 8 a.m. to 9 a.m. the next morning, in case the shift went over twelve hours. I went through the doors and up the stairs into the obstetric wing. I didn't recognise anything. I introduced myself to the registrar, who was on the phone; she gave me a thumbs-up. I folded my paper square. My first job was prescribing some paracetamol on the postnatal ward, which seemed manageable.

After an hour, my bleep went off. I found a phone, and when it answered an ODP asked me if I was the F2. When I said I was, she told me to come to theatre four straight away to assist in a caesarean section. She said *cat one section* in a forceful way. I didn't know what this was, but I guessed it was urgent. I went down to the operating department changing rooms, took my skirt and shirt off and put some scrubs on and some rubber surgical clogs. The clogs were clammy, and I regretted that I hadn't thought to wear socks. I couldn't find theatre four and went through the anaesthetic-only entrance of theatre two by mistake. 'No!' shouted the anaesthetist. When I found the right theatre, I realised it was where I'd had my own emergency caesarean. I scrubbed my fingers and wrists and forearms at the long metal trough in the scrub room and turned the tap off with my elbows. An ODP helped me into a gown, and I picked up the sterile gloves by keeping my fingers inside the sleeve of the gown, as I'd been taught. In theatre, the patient was already on the table with the screen up, and the registrar was painting her abdomen with antiseptic. 'Stand here,' said the reg. 'Hold this, like that; that's it. Just do what I say.' My own abdomen had a numb patch, where the feeling had never come back after the nerves were cut. I could not feel the waistband of my scrub trousers. I looked down at the hill of the patient's abdomen. The registrar started to cut, and I pulled when she told me to pull. As the wound got deeper, my hands filled with the pins and needles of an impending faint.

'Poorly one!' shouted the registrar.

'Sorry,' I said as the ODP pulled me away. She sat me in a chair. 'Put your head down and stay there.'

'No worries, just as long as you don't fall into my field,' said the registrar.

I had never felt faint in theatre before. I looked at the white rubber clogs on my feet. I had taken them from a slot in the changing-room shoe rack. They were labelled with permanent marker: VISI on one foot, TOR on the other.

Soon caesareans became routine, and then, in a now-familiar evolutionary process, they went from routine to annoying. The bleep interrupted and you had to go immediately. On the shelves in the changing room there was only an XXXL top and XXXS trousers and often no clogs in the VISITOR rack at all, which meant purloining someone else's and hoping they didn't notice you walking past with DOCTOR SMITH written on your feet. The operation was quick and usually straightforward; when it wasn't, it was terrible. A baby got stuck with its head in the patient's pelvis and after trying and failing to pull it out, the registrar had to call the consultant in. We waited over the patient's open abdomen, the anaesthetist keeping up a stream of chat with the patient behind the screen, asking her and her husband if they liked football, while the registrar and I stood with our hands folded as though we'd been making pastry, and the theatre staff found jobs and bustled in a representation of normality. The paediatricians had been fast-bleeped to theatre as soon as it was clear there was a problem, and an F2 and a registrar in regular clothes stood next to the empty resuscitaire, waiting for the baby. 'Fuck's sake, come on,' the obstetrics registrar said quietly. On a table in the corner my bleep went off repeatedly and the ODP answered it. 'She's in theatre, you'll have to bleep back. I don't know how long, no.' I couldn't feel my scrub trousers and worried that they were falling down. At last the consultant ran in with his gown open at the back and told the patient to excuse him, he was going to 'dive straight in'. 'Hold this and don't fucking move unless I tell you,' he said to me. He and the registrar groped in the patient's abdomen. 'Move move move move move!' he shouted. At last, the baby swung into the air like a shot rabbit before the paediatricians took it for resuscitation. I never found out if it was all right.

There was more to obstetrics than labour and delivery. We also saw women before and after they'd given birth. Pregnant women came to labour ward triage all day and all night. They thought their waters might have broken. They thought labour might have started. They thought the baby had stopped moving. They had noticed blood. At term, they hoped to be told they were indeed in labour. Pre-term, they hoped to be told that everything was OK. The atmosphere in each room was inflated by the presence of the unborn baby, an extra person silently agitating for help. Other extra people – mothers, friends, partners – interceded, soothed, made jokes and looked at their phones. Once I went into a triage room and the woman's husband was shaving at the sink. 'I've got work in a minute,' he said. It was the F2's job to clerk the arrivals and make a plan for each. Unless it was an emergency, the plan was always 'P: Discuss with senior'.

I had been to triage myself, at thirty-six weeks pregnant, when the baby stopped moving. I lay on the couch with my head full of bleak scenes as the midwife got out the monitor. As she put on the straps, a limb travelled across my abdomen like Jaws's fin. 'Looks like he's woken up,' said the midwife. I feel like an idiot, I said, as all the women did when the trace showed the baby behaving normally. But you were not an idiot if the trace was bad. Then you cursed your own stupidity for not having come sooner, for having tried to wake the baby with cold drinks, fizzy drinks, star jumps, bright light. 'When did you say you last felt him move?'

Any woman admitted to the labour ward had to have a cannula put in, in case anything went wrong, as obstetric emergencies were high speed, and bloody. Obstetrics used massive cannulas, greys, the kind used by super-emergency professionals and helicopter medics. (It takes six minutes to run a litre of fluid through a grey as opposed to twenty-two minutes to get the same volume through a tiny blue one.) 'It's Poiseuille's law, isn't it,' the registrar said. 'Velocity is inversely proportional to the fourth power of the radius, or whatevs.' What? I said. 'The fatter the pipe, the faster the flow.' I was fine at putting in cannulas after two years of constant practice. The plastic tube was packaged with a needle threaded inside it: the tip of the needle protrudes from the end of the tube. To insert one, you found a straight length of vein and pushed the needle in until you saw a little blood flashback into the tube. Then you advanced a tiny bit further, to ensure the end of the cannula was fully inside the vein. Once in, you pulled the needle out backwards while still inching the cannula in. I loved the sensation of the cannula floating off the needle and into the vein. It felt like pushing a sledge over smooth snow, with a little traction but no friction, and I loved how they didn't hurt after the initial stab if you did them correctly; they seemed a mark of competence.

The women usually had easy veins, as you have more blood circulating when you're pregnant. The hospital slang was 'hosepipes'. But when I tried to slip a grey cannula into a hosepipe, it went wrong. I talked too much, allowing the woman too much time to dwell on the size of the cannula. Silence descended. When I poked the cannula in, I got a flashback, but couldn't advance. I kept pushing, even though I knew I shouldn't have to push if I was in the right place. The patient's skin rucked up. 'Be more confident,' the midwife suggested. The next time, I stuck the grey straight in. The vein burst, creating an instant bruise. 'That hurt worse than labour!' the patient said. At home, R offered to let me practise on him. 'But don't miss,' he said. I felt he'd misunderstood the concept of practice. I went to fetch an orange.

As a GP, no one needed me to put in grey cannulas any more, or hold a pair of forceps, or agree that this was a good plan even though I had no understanding of this plan. Mostly, no one was haemorrhaging. I felt that I was wasting learning; there was nowhere to put the obs and gynae knowledge I'd acquired. I could talk to patients about different kinds of birth, and I was better at examination than I had been. But community obstetrics and gynaecology – which we now called 'women's health' – was less straightforward than it had been in hospital. In hospital, things were usually obvious. Even in a foreign country, I'd been able to guess why women were there, what they expected, and what we needed to do next. In labour triage there was a team to help you, and lots of equipment; if you weren't sure what a pain signified, you could 'sit on it', keep the woman in until you were sure, maybe get some blood tests or another CTG trace or a scan. In the community, disaster was hidden. An ectopic pregnancy was just an abdominal pain until you, the doctor, had generated this diagnosis. There were many other diagnoses you could come up with, and no one to tell you that you were wrong, or remind you of the other possibilities. Women didn't necessarily know they were pregnant: you had to think to do a pregnancy test, explain the rationale for the test, gain consent for the test, and then pass on a piece of information that was never without emotional charge. Routine disorders didn't always advertise themselves as gynaecological either, hiding in stories of relationship problems, or turning up as pains in unexpected places.

Every week in GP was full of gynaecology, as women tend to prefer female GPs. Soon I couldn't believe I'd ever struggled in a gynaecology examination room with a powerful lamp and an electronic couch with stirrups and a nurse passing me equipment. Now you had to do everything by yourself, and you used whatever was available in whatever room you found yourself in. 'Flop your knees apart,' I said; 'OK, flop one knee.' The patient's other knee was flush up against the wall. Her clothes were draped over the clinical waste bin. I wheeled out the lamp, creating a trip wire of stretched cable which I stepped over in an experienced way. I shook the kit out on the strip of couch between the patient's legs. 'I'm sorry, it's a bit cramped in here,' I said. 'Don't move your feet because I'm using you as a work surface.' I prepared a blob of lubricant by the patient's left foot and arranged the swabs next to her right foot. 'I always think it must be strange to be a doctor,' she said.

Community gynaecology contained more matter-of-fact weirdness than anything I encountered in hospital. Examining Ms Smith, I found her cervix had a white ring on it like a Polo mint. I had no idea what it was. Eventually she told me she had been reading on the internet about home remedies for vaginal discharge. She had dipped a doughnut hair accessory in bleach and inserted it into her vagina. The ring was a chemical burn. I took out expected foreign bodies (forgotten tampons) and the occasional unexpected foreign body (a new potato). One patient tried to get me to pull her cervix out. She had felt something that she was convinced wasn't supposed to be there, and it was only mid-examination that I realised she had become suspicious of her normal anatomy.

In obs and gynae, sex had been low on the agenda. We asked patients when they'd last had unprotected sex, in order to ascertain the likelihood of pregnancy or infection, but we left it there. Sex was obviously occurring, but we didn't dwell on it. In general practice, we never stopped talking about it. I remembered a lecture from medical school, in which a professor of primary care had described a novel method for investigating erectile dysfunction. It involved wrapping the penis in a paper ring made from the trim from a sheet of stamps. If an erection took place, the power of 'the arousal' – as the professor described it – would tear the perforations, and the patient would wake up to find a fragment of paper in his bed. No erection: ring intact. In retrospect, this should have signalled the improv air of much of community sexual health.

Once I realised that female patients were going to tell me confusing things for ever, I did a postgraduate course in sexual and reproductive health. Four of us attended the theory module: three GPs and a practice nurse. 'What do all human beings have in common?' the consultant asked in his introduction. Need for food? Water? Sleep? 'Sex!' he said. I knew this was specialty bias – a renal specialist would have said 'kidneys!' and a cardiologist 'hearts!' – but even so, I was charmed. 'Even if they don't look like they are, never assume they're not,' he added. 'They'll catch you out.' We each had to say what we hoped to get out of the course. The GPs said, be more confident at managing contraceptive needs in the population etc. The practice nurse said she needed to learn how to put in the contraceptive implant, as by the time her patients received an appointment for the family planning clinic, they were often already pregnant. 'They're quite active, my ladies.'

The trainer passed out some contraceptives for us to look at. There was no sniggering, even when he had us massage a water-filled condom with the wrong kind of lubricant in order to demonstrate what the wrong kind of lubricant could do to condoms. The condom burst and the trainer got wet, which surprised me, as he must have known this would happen. Damn, he said. We examined a plastic pelvis arranged on an electronic couch under a brilliant light. I luxuriated in the absence of legs.

'How are you going to talk about sex?' he asked us. 'What language are you going to use?' I remembered a lecture at medical school where a genito-urinary consultant had suggested we mirror the patient. 'If they prefer to say "butt fuck", you could consider saying "butt fuck" too – it can build rapport.' Currently, I was wondering how I was not going to talk about sex. The blandest consultations kept veering off. A few weeks before, a patient had come in about a rash on her wrists. It looked like dermatitis; I prescribed a steroid cream. 'Odd how it's so symmetrical,' I said. 'I think it's the rope we're using for tying each other at the moment; I wonder if I might be allergic to it,' she said.

Later, a trainer came to the practice to teach me how to fit contraceptive coils. I was by now familiar with the misapprehensions surrounding these – that the coil was a device similar in size and scale to an old bedspring or Zebedee's foot; that they could spear your partner's penis, or scour your insides like a bottle brush; that they pumped you so full of hormones you gained sixteen stone and lost your fertility for ever. Occasionally, a patient would believe me when I suggested that the coil was a reasonable method of contraception for some people and consent to have one fitted.

The trainer was near retirement. He had fifty years of experience and a boyish manner. The patients loved him. 'Any magic moments during the last three weeks?' he twinkled. They immediately told him everything. Not having any; having too many; the magic has gone. 'About seven months ago,' said a forty-three-year-old. 'He thinks that isn't frequent enough. Do you think that's frequent enough?' 'Can you please prescribe me some HRT?' said an eighty-two-year-old, a few days later. 'I have lost interest in having sex with my husband. Masturbation is fine.'

'Are you needing the coil for contraception?' I asked a patient. 'Only accidentally,' she said. 'You're having sex by accident?' 'Essentially, yes,' she said. 'Accidental person, I mean. Accidentally not my spouse.'

I had recently attended a conference about women's health. I had sat in the top tier of a lecture theatre enjoying the feeling of being back at medical school. I longed to write things down in a notebook again. Around me, you could pick out the GPs: tired-looking women in cardigans. Down on the stage, in a pool of light, a gynaecologist in a green dress gave a presentation. What's New in Contraception. Running the pill together so as to erase the seven-day break, 'although that's not actually new, I know we've all been doing that for ages'. We have? said the GP sitting next to me. A coil designed as a string of beads. A microchip implanted in the patient's hip. The GP sighed. It was hard not to envy the specialists their confidence. In one presentation, a microbiologist explained how she had managed to isolate and identify a single strain of multi-drug-resistant gonorrhoea. She knew it had travelled from South-East Asia, and that there was another case in Australia. 'As a microbiologist, I actually love gonorrhoea,' she said. This was certainty in a field that lacked any such thing ordinarily. 'There's no WAY I can be pregnant,' a patient had said to me the week before. 'It's a miracle. Do the test again!'

Sometimes now I had medical students sitting in with me. 'The circle of learning,' said one of the GPs. The presence of students rarely discouraged the patients. Or this is what I thought, until the patients came back later and I discovered their explicit revelation had actually been only partial disclosure, and now they wished to download an even more explicit revelation. The students were confounded by common problems, which I now realised we had barely or never been taught about: the menopause, breastfeeding, anything to do with vaginas, and everything to do with sex.

Occasionally a student would ask some confounding question: what is the molecular biology of immunity? I liked to deflect this by getting a question in first. 'There's a link between sex and heart disease, can you think what it is?' I said. I was thinking of erectile dysfunction, which is sometimes an early warning that the arteries are furring up. Random yet specific questions are the hallmark of medical teaching. Smith was unfazed. 'Sometimes a man has an affair, which is stressful, and they have a lot of sex, which is also stressful, and in the middle of the act he has a heart attack – maybe because of the stress, together with the exercise?' 'Good answer,' I said. I liked to think of myself as encouraging.

Pain

'We haven't talked about the elephant in the room,' the registrar said. I was the F1 on a surgical rotation, and our registrar loved to teach. She had taken us into a side room to instruct us on bowel diseases. 'What do you think the elephant is?' she said. She blew into a latex glove and then twisted one of its fingers to show us how a strictured gut might appear on an X-ray. 'Apple-core sign,' she said. 'Bowel stricture. What else should you be thinking about?' I was confused. Was this an idiom that medicine took literally? How did this relate to the elephant? Was the twisted finger something to do with a trunk? 'It's pain!' she said. 'Pain is the elephant in the room. Of course you have to work out what's wrong and how to make it better. A bit of pinched bowel is probably going to need an operation. But what about the pain? Beware of getting so caught up in solutions that you ignore half of the problem.'

We were taught about pain at medical school. We learnt about pain pathways, and about how the models were inadequate to explain the complexity of what was going on. The sensation of pain had to pass through the brain in order to be interpreted as pain. 'No brain, no pain,' said the lecturer. Sometimes the pain existed *only* in the brain, which didn't make it hurt any less. In phantom limb pain, the brain retains a model of the part that's been lost and continues to report sensations from the missing limb. On the vascular ward, a patient who'd had her leg amputated explained how she could still feel the pain from her foot ulcer, even though it was no longer there. Her foot's other sensations had also continued, including an itch that could not now be scratched. Worst for her was that the missing foot was permanently cold. It was as though her brain knew about the cold tissue bucket and could feel its foot abandoned there, permanently without a sock. It was the kind of detail that my children would have needed to know. 'After the chicken gets its head cut off, can its eyes still see?'

We learnt that painful events could occur without pain. Soldiers ran from the battlefield despite their injuries; people crawled from traffic accidents oblivious to damage. On the news, a stabbing victim reported that the stabbing hadn't hurt; he thought he'd been punched. Medicine couldn't entirely explain what was going on, although we knew the brain released analgesic chemicals, and that it could be distracted into omitting to relay messages.

We incorporated pain into our history-taking. The mnemonic was SOCRATES – Site, Onset, Character, Radiation, Alleviating factors, Timing, Exacerbating factors, Severity. I wrote it in the margin of my notebook to remind me to ask the right things. Twelve years later, I watched the medical students doing the same thing in my clinics; you could see them mouthing *S-O-C-R-A-* to themselves when they got stuck. 'Does anything make it feel worse? Does anything make it feel better?' We learnt what different conditions were supposed to feel like. Nerve pain was 'shooting' or 'electrical'; bone pain was 'dull' or 'aching'; cardiac pain was 'crushing'.

We were told to look as well as listen. If it was pain from angina the patient wouldn't point but rather gesture with their hand or fist, as the heart muscle cannot communicate its precise location. In fact, none of the internal organs gave clear signals; the act of pointing suggested the problem lay more superficially, in the skin or a skeletal muscle. The patient might wave a hand in the air to show pain coming in waves, or clench her fist to show squeezing. Kidney stones created a restless patient who could not lie still. With other pains the patient stayed motionless so as not to agitate the affected part: this was called splinting. Inflammation inside the abdomen made manoeuvres painful. 'Watch them when they get up on the couch,' said the surgical registrar. 'They won't "hop up" if they've got peritonitis.'

On the wards, pain was less noisy than we had expected. They were not full of screams and howls. I stood by a bed as a man put his shirt on after a thoracotomy, and he tensed at each buttonhole but made no sound. If patients did cry out or moan, everyone found it intolerable. The patient or her neighbour would press their buzzer, and if he had no medicine to give, the nurse would bleep the doctor immediately. But we couldn't come immediately. Pain was not a medical emergency – we had to see the patients who were bleeding or septic or unconscious first. On the wards, there was a predictably bleak time at around 4 a.m. when the evening pain-killer ran out. The next regular dose was two hours away. Patients woke up in this ditch and cried for relief. You must write up enough PRN, the medical registrar told us (pro re nata – when necessary), so the nurses have something to give. Don't make people wait. But even if the medication was prescribed, there was delay built into administering opioids. Fetching the drugs was a two-nurse job, one to get the medication and the other to check it. Both had to sign the controlled drug book. The CD cupboard was locked, and only one nurse on each ward had the key.

The intensity of a pain was not an indication of its significance.

A pain could be severe but harmless, as with gout, or labour; or it could be niggling but serious, such as the pain caused by many types of tumour. We learnt to fear painless things: painful jaundice was gallstones; painless jaundice, cancer. A patient's wife came to talk to us about the patient experience of heart disease. I didn't think a heart attack would feel like that, she said. She had noticed her husband kneading his shirt pocket one morning, and then he collapsed. I thought it would have hurt more, she said. Often the hospital patients didn't mention their pain at all, focusing instead on discomforts. The cost of the television, the cost of the parking. The plastic pillow. The too-tight stockings. The room is hot. The tea is cold. When I asked Mr Smith about his recent laparotomy, he said that his stomach had 'caused a bit of bother. But it's settled down now.'

We learnt about pain scales. They were baffling. How could anyone measure what hurt more and what hurt less? Surely you couldn't weigh pain. I thought of my medical school entrance exams, the weighing scale in the lift. But some pains appeared to have achieved exceptionality, acknowledgement that they were especially bad. Arterial ulcers; kidney stones; cluster headache; childbirth. Each specialty also had its own ranking of procedures; the level of pain didn't necessarily correlate with the look of what you were doing. Lung surgery was more painful than hip surgery was more painful than hysterectomy, which was less painful than bunion surgery. A needle in the groin hurt less than the wrist, although it looked more barbaric. On a respiratory job, I assisted with talc pleurodesis, in which sterile talc is instilled into the space around the lungs. The procedure is used to treat pleural effusions, which can occur as a complication of some cancers. The talc creates an irritant reaction, which stops more fluid accumulating. It was a bedside procedure; in fact, an in-bed procedure. The patient lay back on the pillow with her arm behind her head, and the registrar infiltrated some local anaesthetic and then fed the chest drain into the space between the fourth and fifth ribs. When he started to trickle in the chalky fluid, the patient cried out. The pleura are exquisitely sensitive, said the registrar. The patient's face was covered in tears. Exquisitely, when applied to pain, often meant unbearable. We learnt it as a standard description and used it to underline seriousness. You often heard it in handover or referral, where one doctor wished to impress their patient's pain level on another: 'his leg is exquisitely tender'.

I learnt to ask patients to rate their pain. 'If zero is no pain and ten is the worst pain you've ever felt, how would you score your pain today?' I said. Some patients said 'eleven', which undermined their credibility. But more often they were careful over their replies, sometimes reviewing past painful incidents for comparison. 'About eight. No – when I broke my wrist that was an eight. Seven.' Sometimes people seemed to be asking me how bad the pain was, as if they wanted it corroborated. 'About six?' There was a separate scale for children, or anyone who struggled with numbers: the faces pain scale. This featured a cartoon face that started at zero, labelled 'No Hurt'. In increments the face's mouth turned down and its eyebrows moved up. Finally it was distorted with sadness, tears rolling out of its eyes: 'Hurts Worst'. Hurts Worst was ten on ten. I found it hard to look at the Hurts Worst face; the idea that things could get this bad, and that the patient would not be able to tell anyone, was terrible.

Both the pain scales and our mnemonics were inadequate for capturing pain. One day I was cleaning a window at home. As I wiped the cloth near a crack in the glass I had a thought of the kind that comes before an accident: That looks sharp. Patients had often told me these thoughts. 'That looks steep'; 'that looks unstable'; 'this is going a bit fast': each thought related afterwards, from inside a neck collar, bandages, a cast. A moment later, I'd cut my thumb. A ridiculous fan of blood sprayed the window. I looked at my thumb to make sure it was still attached, and when I saw it was, I felt carefree. The pain came after a short delay. It had a surprising quality of warmth, from the blood dripping out. About four on ten? It was easy to characterise and grade this small pain from a harmless injury. Site: thumb, onset: just now, character: throbbing.

But most pains didn't cooperate like this. I remembered the accident I'd had when I was fourteen, during a school trip to Greece. Our coach arrived at a hotel, and we all jumped off and raced up to our rooms. When I opened the door of mine, I saw it had a balcony. I ran out to have a look and went through a closed French window. I hadn't seen it, and the noise of breaking glass was a big surprise. The glass cut my legs and face. I backed up to the sink and spat out blood and looked in the mirror. There was blood everywhere, even running out of my ear. Had I somehow burst my eardrum? It didn't hurt. A taxi came to take me to the hospital, but that hospital sent me on to a bigger hospital that had an X-ray machine. Everything began to hurt during the second taxi ride. A doctor sewed up my face and legs – my ear was fine – while the taxi driver stood next to my head. 'Be brave! That's it, my brave!' he said, kissing my forehead. The next days were dominated by the diesel smell of the coach as we finished the tour. It was hard to get off with bandaged legs, so I mostly stayed in my seat and looked at Greece through the window.

I relived the accident to myself for months afterwards, reconstructing events, recalling more images: the glass spikes protruding from the frame of the window and the triangular shards on the floor, the balcony with its red geraniums, the pool of blood in the sink. But the pain had gone. I couldn't re-experience it, describe it or score it. You know what they say about childbirth, a patient said to me: you can't remember the pain.

During my own first labour, the midwife came to ask me if I had pain. Six on ten? I said. I waited for her to tell me if I'd got it right. Later a registrar came and started a Syntocinon drip to speed things up, and now the contractions came in the famous waves. But they were like a wave of unreasonable size and force that had once picked me up in the sea and smashed me down on my head. A number didn't seem sufficiently dimensional to express characteristics of force and volume, or the sensation of lost control. A minute lasted for a long time, and then came again sooner than a minute. I couldn't keep a tab on the hours. Although I couldn't feel the sensations again afterwards, I could recall all of these features. The pain scales missed out so much, including what pain did to time – the damaged minutes, the amplification of days.

The Canadian psychologist Ronald Melzack realised the shortcomings of pain scales when he was a postgraduate student in the 1970s. His book *The Puzzle of Pain* describes his research. He started to collect 'pain words': words that patients used to describe pain. He worked with his research subjects to allocate each pain word a relative intensity. 'Shooting' was found to represent more pain than 'flashing', which in turn implied more pain than 'jumping'. Along with another psychologist, Warren S. Torgerson, he created the McGill Pain Questionnaire, in which seventy-eight words were grouped into themes including temporal ('beating', 'pounding'), spatial ('jumping', 'shooting'), thermal ('scalding', 'searing'), fear ('frightful', 'terrifying') and punishment ('gruelling', 'cruel', 'vicious'). The questionnaire helped patients to capture pain in a deeper way, by acknowledging its emotional and psychological aspects. It was too time-consuming to use on the wards or in clinic, but it was now in my mind when I asked people for numbers. And – acknowledging to myself the impossibility of reconciling 'vicious' and 'pounding' on a one-to-ten scale – I now rarely asked for numbers at all.

This was also because pain was different in the community. As a GP, I saw less acute pain and more chronic pain, pain that was hard to put on any kind of scale. It often lacked an obvious source, and it could less often be fixed. By definition, it didn't go away. Patients came with a complaint they described as 'too much pain', which would have confounded Melzack: every part of their bodies radiated a different discomfort. There was nothing to see – no cut, no bruise, no deformity. For the first time, I realised the advantages of looking ill, of having a rash, bruising, a cast, crutches. If you intrigued other people, you could expect to be shown interest and concern. 'Are you ill? What did you do? Did it hurt?' People asked questions out of sympathy, but also in the hope of hearing a story, ideally one where suffering met resolution. These were the kinds of stories I liked too, that I'd read in childhood. Disaster! Relief! I was reading Solzhenitsyn's *Cancer Ward* in part just to find out what was going to happen to everyone. Would Ludmila Dontsova, the doctor, recover after her own cancer diagnosis? Sometimes at the practice, I heard the patients talking in the waiting room. 'Rushed to hospital'; 'Touch and go'; 'The doctor said if I'd waited another hour ...'

By contrast, the chronic pain patient looked fine, but was alone in a room with an elephant. I knew doctors didn't ask enough about pain, but neither did anyone else. The patients were lonely, estranged by their suffering. This was pain without climax or resolution or moral or point, and it made a poor story.

Old ailments like sciatica and osteoarthritis had been joined by other hard-to-treat problems – fibromyalgia, CFS-ME, POTs, hypermobility, seronegative arthritis. There was pain everywhere, all over the body, in every muscle and bone. Or there was pain in one structure – the abdomen, the pelvis, one ear, one knee – that never revealed its cause but never remitted. Unhappy histories accompanied these pains: delay to diagnosis, unsympathetic clinicians, controversial pathology. The patients could not accept the failure of medicine to reduce their suffering. 'I can't go on like this,' Mrs Smith said. 'Something has to be done.' They brought their disappointment to the consultation along with their distress. Pain was a signal that something was wrong, so what was wrong, and why hadn't we fixed it? It was a sensible belief: we all knew that pain carried messages. Patients with acute problems – a sore shoulder, a painful ankle – often omitted painkillers before their appointment for exactly this reason, so as not to obscure any signs that the doctor might need to interpret.

We too had learnt that pain could be meaningful or give useful information. 'Listen to the pain as well as making the patient comfortable,' said the *Oxford Handbook*. It meant: don't forget about the strictured bowel in your focus on the pain – while the surgeon had urged us not to forget pain in our focus on the stricture. The *OHCM* reminded us that pain could be protective. Skin that lacked sensation was at risk of injury. If the diabetic didn't feel the splinter in her numb foot, she wouldn't know to remove it – the start of the road to sepsis and amputation. Patients with sensory loss were at risk of pressure ulcers. Without pain you had no signal to remove yourself from trouble. It's very hot, it will hurt, I said to the children as I ran the bath. H stuck his hand in the water anyway and took it straight back out. 'Hot!' he said. He was hurt and also angry. 'I told you it was hot,' I said, wondering if a good parent would be scoring this point. It was easy to learn the acute pain lesson: make it stop. But in chronic pain, the messages were useless, reinforcing responses that made the situation worse, enforcing immobility and generating fear.

Mrs Smith had had fibromyalgia for six years. She walked with a cane that she had purchased for herself after an NHS physio-therapist had tried to explain she didn't need one. She spent the nights on her laptop trying to solve the problem. Medicine didn't know shit and didn't give a shit, she told me. I couldn't say she was wrong: we had failed to make her better. I was familiar with the forums and their theories. Has your doctor checked you for deficiencies in vitamin B12, D, K? Have they offered you pre-gabalin, gabapentin, amitriptyline, fentanyl? You need an MRI of your brain, your neck, your spine. There were many conspiracy theories, and they were comforting, providing explanations that we had failed to give, a rationale where there was otherwise only a daily experience of futility. What kind of useless story had someone crippled by endless pain, for no apparent reason, with no apparent cause, and offered no remedy or redemption? Medicine was withholding information, investigation, medication; we had interests in making people worse.

It was true: on occasion, medicine *had* made people worse. Bulgakov made himself worse in this way. He was injured while serving as a doctor in the First World War, or perhaps he had a reaction to a diphtheria vaccine – no one seems to know where his pain came from. He treated himself with morphine. In *A Country Doctor's Notebook*, there is a story called 'Morphine', in which the doctor is called Sergei Polyakov. 'I must give due praise to the man who first extracted morphine from poppyheads. He was a true benefactor of mankind. The pain stopped 7 min after the injection,' Polyakov tells us. He asks the nurse for the keys to the dispensary, so he can get more of the drug. A clinic in early-twentieth-century Russia has a CD cupboard just like our own. Soon Polyakov is addicted, and each paragraph of the story is a craving for the next paragraph, which contains the next fix. When chemists analysed Bulgakov's manuscripts fifty years later they found morphine molecules all over the pages.

Doctors are still facilitating opioid addiction now. By the time I was fully qualified, we knew these drugs didn't work for chronic pain. The patients developed tolerance, and then dependence; the drugs stopped working. Trying to explain that these medicines didn't work for 'this kind' of pain neglected every aspect of pain except its number on a one-to-ten scale. Maybe they didn't treat pain, but they did ameliorate the despair, obscure the slowness of the minutes, blot out some of the futility. 'It does fuck all. But I give less of a fuck,' Mr Smith said, when I asked how his morphine was working. He was on a fentanyl patch, with oral morphine for 'breakthrough pain'. Two years previously, he had had an operation on his spine to take out a protruding disc. Before the operation, his pain was 9/10; after the operation, his pain was 9/10. The disc was gone, but the pain was no better – a recognised outcome of some spinal surgeries. I remembered the months as this fact sank in: it wasn't going to get better. Every time I saw his name on my screen, I felt a premonition of the coming disappointment. The surgeons had betrayed him, the doctors had betrayed him. They had drawn a picture that made sense and proposed a solution that made sense; now nothing made sense. He was on too much opioid analgesia, and every appointment was an argument.

'I'm worried you've become addicted,' I said.

'Fucking right I'm addicted. I don't care,' he said. 'You can't leave me in pain.'

'It's dangerous.'

'I don't give a fuck.'

When I was training, we had learnt that there was an epidemic of pain, and that we had failed to treat it adequately due to fears of causing addiction. The patients shared these fears. I spent much of my time trying to get people to accept analgesia; opioids were essential in cancer pain, and they were fundamental to good palliative care. The feeling at large then was that we had not unlocked the CD cupboard often enough. We should be using opioids more freely and worrying less about addiction. The pain 'mops up' the addicting effects of the drug, a lecturer told us; you won't become addicted if you're using it for the right indication. The American Pain Society called pain 'the fifth vital sign'; they wanted it added to the observations, so that you would have four parameters you could count (pulse, respiratory rate, temperature, oxygen saturations) and one that the patient counted for you; we would add his observation of himself. The good news was this observation could be treated. Opioid addiction rates increased largely through the work of the family doctors, as GPs are called in the States: they saw most of the chronic pain, and therefore issued most of the prescriptions.

Unpicking this mistake became a dismal feature of some consultations. It destabilised my tentative understanding of what doctors were for. I knew that medicine had always dissembled, and doctors had always got things wrong. Historical treatments were at best useless, at worst harmful. Doctors had used turpentine for cholera, mercury for syphilis, leeches for croup. Doctors spread infection on postnatal wards and refused to believe Ignaz Semmelweis, the Hungarian physician who pioneered antisepsis, when he suggested that medical students should be washing their hands between handling cadavers and delivering babies. We were in error even when we weren't making actual errors, through our promotion of facts that turned out to be no such thing: encouraging smoking, prescribing cough medicine containing morphine. I thought of Somerset Maugham's mother, whose doctor prescribed pregnancy as a treatment for her tuberculosis. She died six days after the delivery of her sixth child. Even now, when we had a scientific justification for most things that we did, every medicine we prescribed still had the potential to cause harm.

I had been taught that we based our medical treatments on evidence: on scientific interrogation of what worked and what didn't. In medical school, we had learnt how to appraise evidence, how to read a paper, how to look for bias or distortion. Since medical school, the number of papers I read had gone down as the workload increased. I took my evidence on trust – from the medical journals or national guidance. I knew evidence could shift as research progressed. Now I learnt that evidence could be wrong, and worse, a conspiracy theory could be correct. There was an opioid epidemic in America and the UK, and the manufacturers of OxyContin were accused of misleading doctors deliberately, downplaying the addictiveness of the medicines and encouraging prescribing.

In clinic I had to try to separate people from the medication we had given them. I tried to remember if I'd started any patients on strong opioids. I often gave people weaker ones such as codeine. I had ticked repeat scripts without interrogating the prescription any further. Now we started to look. But you couldn't just stop prescribing the medicine: the patients were addicted, and you had to bring them in to the surgery for what you billed as a conversation and they saw as an attack. We now know these drugs don't work very well for this kind of pain, I explained, directly contradicting whoever had started the tablet.

I had felt more convincing as a doctor at the age of eight, when I'd given my teddy his water injection. But with training, I had grown more uncertain even as I tried to work on my tolerance of uncertainty. Not only had doctors made things worse instead of better, but we had now lost an option for treatment. Pain was a recurring theme in consultation, but the top of the analgesia ladder had been sawn off.

I tried to step back, to put a space between myself and the pain, to resist the desire to fix it immediately. I remembered an afternoon at medical school. The consultant teaching us had stuck her arm out as I'd gone towards a patient's bed. 'Start further back,' she'd said, steering me away with her arm. 'Use the end of the bed as a marker. Stand behind it for a moment, take everything in.' I had recently read an essay about medicine in history. With the invention of the stethoscope, the doctor moved away from his patient, said the author of the essay. Before it, to hear anything, he needed to press his ear directly against the chest. Now he could keep some distance. Without a bed frame to show me where to stand, I was finding you could use the professional manner like a length of stethoscope tubing to create a flexible distance between your listening ear and your patient's inmost heart.

You had to be close enough to feel but distant enough to retain the ability to think. A manner, a persona, was helpful in this; once in role, the distance between me and the patient was dictated by our parts. But role-playing brought its own concerns. One day, consulting, I heard myself give a gurgling, fruity laugh, the sort of laugh that I associated with the legendary GPs of the golf course. Would I be going home in a shiny car, my leather case at my side? Was I now one of literature's doctors, learned in condescension?

I spoke full medical English now, both registers. I addressed children as poppet and babies as sweetpea, and since I'd worked in the north of England I had been calling patients darling, although I'd tried to wind this down now I was back in the south. I made standard jokes. 'Has he been misbehaving again?' I asked the patient's partner.

Hop up on there and let's have a look at you, I would say. Let's have a feel, let's have a listen. I noticed I was phrasing everything as 'us'; perhaps I was asking my patients for help, trying to signal that we were in this together. The *OHCM* urged compassion for everyone. Understanding that some doctors might not know what this was, it supplied a definition. 'Imaginative indwelling into another's condition,' it said. But how was I to indwell and outdwell thirty times in ten hours, and stay at the right distance overall? How to avoid catching all the pain without becoming a machine? I thought of Kapa, the wife of the patient Nikolayevich in *Cancer Ward*. 'Doctors are a detestable race, anyway. How dare they talk about production achievement when it's living people they're processing?'

I tried to identify what the patient wanted as I greeted him in the waiting room. I wanted to know if any elephants were coming in with him. Come on through, I said, as we walked down the corridor together. Take a seat. Once he'd sat down, I looked to see if he moved closer or was edging away. Was he ill or well, comfortable or unsettled? Did he want a diagnosis or was he here for a prescription? How much of this consultation was going to be about pain?

The days continued to mix banality and alarm. One lunchtime I visited an eighty-year-old man. His son had phoned to say he was breathing fast. I left the surgery as soon as I could. When I got to the house, Mr Smith's wife opened the door as I reached for the handle. 'I saw you coming up the path,' she said. She led me into their sitting room. Her husband was sitting on the sofa, hands on his knees, breathing at thirty breaths a minute which was easy to count as each breath made a noise. I knew he needed an ambulance as soon as I saw him, but I made myself get the information first. The wife and the son told me the history and I knelt in front of Mr Smith to check his observations. 'I'm going to phone an ambulance, bear with me,' I said to his wife. They nodded. I went to the kitchen to phone 999. 'Tell me exactly what has happened,' said the operator. They always said this, and I always thought that if I could do it I would have fulfilled the goal of my life. I told the operator I was a GP. 'Does this condition present an immediate threat to life?' said the operator. 'It does, yes,' I said. I looked at the mugs on the mug tree. World's Best Mum, World's Best Dad and World's Best Son. When I came back, there was a travel bag on the floor, and Mrs Smith was helping her husband into his jacket. His eyes looked panicked. He raised a finger to acknowledge my return. 'That was quick!' I said, indicating the bag. 'Best to keep one packed, at our age. I've got one too,' said Mrs Smith. She was holding a kitchen roll in her hands; she tore off two sheets and put one into each of her husband's pockets. She didn't speak to him but tucked the tissues in carefully. He watched everything she was doing. The window filled up with the white shape of the ambulance, and the son went to open the door.

Three paramedics came in. 'GP's still here!' one said. 'Miracle!' They stood together, studying Mr Smith on the sofa. Paramedics never look worried: it's a requirement of the job that you never betray fear or anxiety. Sometimes their absolute calm reminded me of a surgical joke I'd seen on the internet.

> Never say 'whoops!', say 'there'.
> Usage: 'There. I've severed the aorta.'

My doctor job was to convey anxiety to them, to justify the 999 call and the need for urgency. I handed over, emphasising the breathing, the oxygen saturations below 80, and the patient's blue fingers. It sounded needy. 'OK, we can take it from here, thank you,' the paramedic said. 'Don't want to keep you from your busy day.'

Back in the surgery, I saw a rash, a cough, a back pain, an anxious mood, a swollen leg, a vaginal discharge, a pain all over, a headache, a pelvic pain, a mole, a depression, another depression, and a fever. I never detached patients from their symptoms any more; I made this list as an experiment, to try out a form of distance, to see if I could re-establish an objective method. It wasn't possible; the thirteen people still entered the room before their problems, and I had failed once again to work algorithmically, and I was once again running late.

The second depressed patient barely spoke and wouldn't meet my eye. I looked away from him to allow him space to lift his gaze. His despair felt like dislike. When I asked him if he was hurting himself, he said he was; when I asked to see, he pulled up his sleeve to show me twenty or so cuts up his arm. Shall we get those dressed? I suggested. He declined. He was not suicidal 'at the moment', he said. Have you written a suicide note? I asked, despising myself as I always did. It felt more glibly invasive than any physical examination. I'm going to contact the crisis mental health team, I said. With your permission. 'You're the doctor,' he said.

The fever belonged to an eight-year-old. He also had a rash, and his observations were abnormal. He looked pale, but his lips were red and his eyes were bloodshot. I phoned the hospital to ask if they'd accept him, and typed a letter for his mother to take with them. '5+ days fever + rash ?Kawasaki' I typed at the end of the letter; a rare but serious vascular disease. I didn't think he had it, but in this ten minutes I couldn't say for sure that he didn't. His mother watched me typing. Her son laid his head in her lap. Are you OK to drive him there? I asked. It'll be quicker than getting an ambulance. I thought of the paramedics standing in Mr Smith's sitting room and wondered whether Mr Smith had died. I felt bad that I was filling up the hospital with patients, with my patients, whose difficulties I was powerless to fix. I thought of the literary doctors who'd come apart: the useless Dr Bovary; the idealistic Dr Lydgate in *Middlemarch*. 'He always regarded himself as a failure; he had not done what he once meant to do.'

Patients came for many reasons other than pain. Sometimes they were ill, but more often they wanted to confirm that they weren't. They wanted a diagnosis, an explanation, advice, reassurance, medication, a plan, a letter or a note. Or they just wanted their symptoms documented, which was fine, as it was my job to write everything down. I left the notes open but tried not to look at them during the consultation, mindful of all the videos I'd been shown during my training in which the doctor looked at the computer rather than at the patient, and the patient twitched, and we all felt we could do it better. You can't hide behind the screen, one of the lecturers had said during medical school. Want to bet, said the student next to me. Occasionally, patients told me what I should put, or asked me to leave something out. I am not allowed to omit anything, I said. I meant *intentionally*. The notes were all omission, as I had to complete them in thirty-five seconds. I wrote a Hx/Ex/Ix/P and used my own invented shorthand for anything else. I typed 'adv' for advised, 'disc' for discussed, 'sug' for suggested. I read the phrases of my colleagues. 'Reassurance given.' 'Explored concerns.' Sometimes I recorded a pain score. A high score helped justify a hospital admission; a low score made me feel better about having sent the patient home. Sometimes, lost for where to go next, I resurrected the golden minute and found it worked after all. People would fill any gap if you left them one.

The Cure for Good Intentions

'Someone has definitely said the Q-word,' my colleague said. The practice was meeting to discuss the novel coronavirus; so far, we had concluded that chaos was coming. We sat together in our small staff room, drinking coffee and inhaling each other's breath. It was still early in the pandemic, and we didn't know much. I loved medicine's embrace of superstition. Full moon meant difficult night shift. Bed thirteen spelt death. One hospital I worked in omitted the thirteenth floor entirely: the lift went 12th floor–14th floor, and no one said a thing. The first thing you learnt in hospital was never to use the word quiet, as to do so would incite a hurricane of admissions and arrests.

Emails about Covid were arriving hourly. They came from Public Health England, the British Medical Association, the General Medical Council, the Royal College of General Practitioners, the Clinical Commissioning Group and the Local Medical Committee. Each contained new instructions and what we immediately learnt to call SOPs (standard operating procedures). Next day another email would arrive, revising the previous instructions and SOPs. See patients with fever in a 'red zone'. See other patients in a 'yellow zone'. Wear an apron, mask and gloves for all patients. Wear an apron, mask, gloves and visor for all patients. Have your patient count to thirty to assess their oxygen level over the phone. Do not have your patient count to thirty to assess their oxygen level over the phone. Prepare to palliate your patients at home as there will be no room in the hospital. Prepare to run out of palliative drugs and oxygen. Contact this list of patients and tell them they should shield. Contact this other list of patients and tell them the instruction to shield was a mistake.

We set to learning the new disease whose mode of presentation was uncertain and which no one had diagnosed before. We tried to become expert in the new terminology. We coded our consultations in the notes, conscious of collecting data in a live experiment, although *severe acute respiratory syndrome coronavirus 2* was such a lengthy phrase that when you selected it from the software's drop-down list you couldn't initially see what variant of the problem you were picking: 'suspected', 'diagnosed' or 'severe illness due to'.

The early days of the pandemic soon seemed vintage. I remembered when Public Health England first sent us posters to stick on the practice's front door. Have you recently visited Wuhan Province in China, or any of these regions of northern Italy: Lombardy, Emilia-Romagna, Veneto, Piedmont or Marche? asked the poster. There was even a map with the dangerous bits of China and Italy shaded in blue, in case you weren't sure where you'd been. The innocence of those notices, with their belief in containability. In northern Italy, we later learnt, GPs had spread the virus through making home visits to the elderly, like Semmelweis's medical students spreading puerperal fever through the wards.

Soon the receptionists put different posters on the door, with graphics of the coronavirus looking like a spiky rubber massage ball. The poster said, in a polite way, DO NOT COME IN. We locked the doors, as we had been instructed. Now everyone thought we were closed. In fact, in some ways we were more open than we had been previously. We were certainly more available, as we spoke to every patient on the same day, where previously the wait was weeks. We were told to triage everyone by phone and only bring in those who needed examination. You had to work out for yourself where your triage boundaries lay: a new level of risk. At medical school they had told us that eighty per cent of the diagnosis is in the history. Now we often aimed for a hundred per cent.

At home scraps of phone calls replayed themselves constantly, as I tried to work out what I might have missed. My head felt like a call centre. I could not read a book or watch television as I needed to keep my brain free for this replay; at the same time the replay made me tired. At work I sat on my chair and watched the list creeping down the screen as each new call was added. Back home I lay on the sofa and immediately opened Twitter. It was like jumping into a swimming pool and having the water blot out noise. I could still consume hundreds of individual people's words, which was the only thing I felt I should be doing, but at least now the voices didn't make a sound.

Everyone in the country was learning acronyms with us: WFH, PPE. Eventually boxes arrived containing gloves and masks and aprons. 'Wouldn't you think a virus could get round the edges of these?' asked the registrar, pulling an apron off the roll. The aprons clung to themselves and it took discipline not to lick your fingers to separate them. A new consignment arrived. 'These are bin liners!' said the nurse. R's practice had scrubs donated by some of the patients, who had sewn them together from old sheets and duvet covers. 'These ones are so soft,' said

R, pulling on a set covered in smiling crocodiles. Was this the right attire for a pandemic, I wondered. Twitter was full of Italian medical staff with PPE-related friction burns on their faces. 'Why not?' he said.

Soon there were forty or fifty phone calls a day. Suicidal; fever; wart; chest pain; dizziness; anxiety; short of breath; rash. Sore knee; sore shoulder; sore throat. Long-term illnesses hadn't gone away; people still rang about their diabetes, bowel disease, dementia and Parkinson's. They had coughs that they thought might be Covid, and coughs that they thought were definitely not Covid. How do you know it's not, I asked. 'I know my body,' Mrs Smith said. My ears popped. At the end of the day I cycled back through the empty streets worrying that I might be stopped by the police and have to justify my outing. I did not want to explain I was a key worker in case someone came and evaluated how key my work was. Trying to work out how ill someone was over the phone was stressful, and reassuring someone they were not ill was a different kind of stressful, but neither activity amounted to anything to be congratulated for, I didn't think, and this was the congratulatory time for the NHS in Britain. The worst was when I arrived home at the same time as the clap, the chorus of applause and pot-banging along our street, as it looked like I was doing a victory lap. Sometimes I ran into our house to get a pan and ran out again to join in, but then I just looked like I was applauding myself.

Some patients needed an examination. Sometimes I brought patients into the building; sometimes, if they had a fever or a cough, I saw them in the car park, or the side alley. In the neighbouring building's yard two women lay on sun loungers. One raised a small dumbbell above her head in a languid way. 'Is it a pandemic or is it a *fundemic*?' said one of the nurses. 'Come round the back,' I explained to patients on the phone, 'and I'll come out to you.' I opened the back door to find the patient standing in the alley near the bins. Sometimes there was a smell of cigarette smoke and sometimes a smell of marijuana, drifting over from the house next door. 'It's not me,' I said, when my eye met the patient's and I saw we were both noticing. I balanced my blood pressure cuff on the windowsill and asked her to relax.

When the patients got Covid it was hard to work out how ill they were. Some people made groaning noises, but the patients who said they didn't want any fuss were more worrying. 'Not breathless over the phone,' I typed. 'Completing whole sentences.' One lunchtime I cycled out to see an infected family at home. I put alcohol gel and an apron and gloves in my bike basket. I had put my oxygen probe in a plastic laboratory sample bag, and my thermometer in another bag. I was pleased the lab bags had HAZARD printed on them: it seemed the most professional part of my amateur operation. On the way there was a soundtrack from hundreds of sparrows in the hedges next to the railway line, and then I realised that they were always there and I was only hearing them now because the city was so quiet.

At the family's house I stood on their front path to put on my apron and mask and gloves. I rang the doorbell and immediately backed away, like an Amazon delivery driver. I interviewed each person in turn about how they were feeling. I watched their chests to see how hard they were breathing and looked at their lips to see if they were blue. Then I threw the sats probe into the hall and showed them how to measure their oxygen levels. After that I threw the thermometer in for them to measure their temperatures. The son, a man in his twenties, threw everything back into my bike basket after they'd finished. 'Score!' he said. The observations are OK, I said, you can stay here for now.

The care home was also closed. To visit, I stood outside and talked with the manager at the door. Then everyone was doing video-calling. I called to speak with Mrs Smith, who was 'more drowsy than usual'. The carer's face filled my screen, and then I was looking at familiar carpet as we walked down the corridor together. She opened a door and pointed the iPad into the room, where Mrs Smith was asleep in a chair. 'Can we go a bit nearer?' I said. She held the tablet up to Mrs Smith's face. 'Mrs Smith, it's the doctor on the video for you!' she said. Mrs Smith moaned. 'Hello, Mrs Smith, it's the doctor!' I said. I was automatically shouting, as though I was actually visiting the care home, where we often shouted. Mrs Smith moaned again and nuzzled her head into the wing of her chair. A smile went over her face like a baby having a dream. 'Can you hear me?' I yelled. 'I don't think she can hear you,' said the carer. 'Actually, she seems a bit better.' 'But she's drowsy?' I said. 'In fact, she's asleep.' 'She's always asleep,' said the carer. 'But now she seems happy asleep. Earlier she seemed – less happy asleep. Not her usual sleeping self.'

One time the receptionist came to say she'd seen Mr Smith walking down the road outside and he didn't look well. All the staff knew Mr Smith. He had a learning disability, and would drop in without an appointment. He would sit on a chair in the waiting room and chat with the receptionists, and then leave saying that a visit to the doctor always made him feel better.

'Do you want to fetch him in, and I'll look at him?' I asked the receptionist. 'Better put him in the red zone.' The red zone was my colleague's consulting room, with extra packets of Clinell wipes. I put on my apron. 'Yikes, what has happened to you?' I said when I saw his thin face. He was wrapped in his coat; when I asked him to take it off I saw that his clothes were too big.

'Are you hungry? What have you been eating?' I said.

'The cafés are shut,' said Mr Smith.

'Can you not cook?' I said, realising this was a stupid question as soon as I asked it. 'Microwave meals?'

'I can't do the microwave. Or the kettle. It's OK, I have crisps,' he said, and gave me a thumbs-up.

I explained I was going to phone a nice social worker for him. I hoped they would be nice; I thought their working life was likely terrible at the moment. 'Do you want tea and biscuits in the waiting room?' I suggested. 'It's outdoors now. New arrangement.'

Whenever I came out of my consulting room the actual waiting room was empty. It looked old-fashioned, with its piles of magazines and posters about Managing Your Asthma and What Is Hypertension? 'Coughs and sneezes spread diseases!' said a poster stuck to the door. The silent radio sat on a table under its sign, This Radio Is On For Your Privacy. Although I missed what we now called face-to-face and transcribed as F2F, I didn't miss the pressure of the full waiting room, which was after all just a square-shaped queue. Phone consulting had ended the ten-minute appointment. We didn't – we couldn't – give precise times for call-backs, and now I could spend four extra minutes assessing a patient without having to look into fourteen disappointed faces afterwards.

Suddenly you could send and receive text messages from the patient's notes. For NHS general practice, only just over the fax, this was an IT revolution. Patients sent photographs of their rashes and their joints and their throats, and we discouraged them from sending images of their genitals. Sometimes people added tape measures or ten-pence pieces to give an idea of scale. It was encouraging how quick and resourceful people were. One man sent a picture of himself holding up a cat, to show what had scratched him.

Occasionally I made video calls, but most of the appointments were on the phone. I took some calls through my headset, so that the patient's voice went directly into my ears, and some on speaker so that my room filled with sound. But I couldn't seem to calibrate my ears. In the practice we wore masks, and every time the GP registrar spoke I looked at him intensely to show I was interested in what he was saying, because I mostly couldn't hear it. For a long time I had found hearing things difficult and now I was finding it very difficult.

Eventually I went to see an audiologist. I paid: I couldn't face phoning a GP in the middle of a pandemic, a phrase we kept saying to each other whenever anything mildly irritating occurred, such as a patient failing to acknowledge that his fungal nail might be OK to wait a few weeks for treatment. 'In the middle of a pandemic!' we said. I purchased an appointment, and no doubt vaulted a massive queue, which made me feel ashamed. I was nonetheless excited to see how private healthcare worked. At the appointment, the audiologist came to fetch me from my car. When I rolled down the window, she pointed a thermometer at my forehead, misted my hands with alcohol spray, and then handed me a new surgical mask *on a tray*. What could we take from this, I wondered. It all seemed so under control. Having my hands misted by someone else felt like attending a spa.

One of the audiology tests was to pick a single voice out of a crowd of voices, and say what the voice had said. It was a familiar problem. Afterwards the audiologist said she could tell I had been concentrating because I was frowning. She offered me some silvery hearing aids 'to match your hair', and so in one sentence I aged twenty years. I was distressed to learn it cost twice as much to be deaf in both ears as to be deaf in one ear. How much I didn't know about the problems people lived with; really, I knew nothing at all.

Wearing the hearing aids increased my sense of fraudulence. Now I felt I was claiming deaf privilege while being insufficiently deaf, to go with being a heroic frontline worker while being insufficiently heroic. Soon I would be accepting vaccine gratitude, without actually vaccinating anyone.

We all had to study the vaccine SOPs when they arrived. Each vial contains six doses. Each dose is 0.3ml. Invert the vial ten times before dilution. Dilute with 1.8ml sodium chloride 0.9% solution. 'The vaccine should not be transported by motor vehicle away from the site of dilution,' the SOP advised. I imagined GPs loading their vehicles and motoring into the sunset.

But I didn't give any vaccinations yet. With the staff we had available it was more useful for me to continue consulting, however useful that was. The medical students had been permitted to return to university; they came to watch me make telephone calls. A seventy-year-old man rang up to say he had been having diarrhoea, and now he had a pain in his belly. Another abdo pain, I told the students. This week everyone had abdominal pain. The week before it had been ankles; eventually it had dawned on me that the gym-goers were having to run on tarmac. I asked Mr Smith to come in for an examination and asked if he would mind seeing a student too. 'We all have to learn,' said Mr Smith. I was grateful to have a real-life patient to share.

The student pressed over Mr Smith's abdomen with his hand and then listened with his stethoscope. 'I can detect no masses and no organomegaly and the abdomen is soft non-tender,' he said. 'May I have a feel?' I asked Mr Smith.

Mr Smith's abdomen was not tender, but I didn't think it was soft – one part was hard, and I could feel the edge of his liver, which you can't usually feel, and that was also hard. 'Have another little prod here,' I said to the student, showing him where to put his hand. Mr Smith raised his head to see what we were doing. 'Can you put your head down, or it makes your tummy a bit tense, due to all your muscles working?' I said.

'I need to ask the hospital to have a look at you,' I told Mr Smith. 'I'm going to use the urgent pathway and ask them to see you as soon as possible.' I waited for a second. 'There is a small chance of something nasty, like cancer,' I said. You always had to tell patients if you wanted to investigate them for cancer. Because that was the ethical thing to do, but also because the hospital was prone to sending out appointment letters headed CANCER INVESTIGATION CLINIC. Mr Smith didn't want to go to the hospital in case he caught Covid. We discussed how clean and careful they were in the radiology department. 'Their PPE is better than ours!' said the student.

The next week Mr Smith's CT report was in my inbox. He had tumours in his liver that might be metastases. I waited for the hospital letter to explain more. When it came, the specialist now thought these were a particular kind of cancer, and that the prognosis, although uncertain, wasn't as bad as it might have been. I phoned Mr Smith to say I was sorry. He was impressed with the hospital. 'They were so clean!' he said. 'I put gel on five times!' I'm sorry about your diagnosis, I said again.

'I knew something wasn't right. Any rate – it could be worse. You should tell your student that.' What should I tell him? I asked.

'It could be worse,' he said. This was one of my new favourite phrases too – along with one day at a time and onwards and upwards. I did have cliché standards; during the first lockdown I'd seen a poster in a window that said 'Try to be a Rainbow in Someone Else's Cloud'. I felt I was more likely to be a lightning bolt, or perhaps sleet. I had learnt, at least, that medicine was not about finding new ways to express yourself, or how nicely you could put together a sentence. It was about trying to understand what others meant, not just the words they said.

Acknowledgements

This book grew out of a column I wrote for *FT Weekend Magazine*, for which I owe great thanks to Liz Jobey, Alice Fishburn and Sue Matthias. Thanks to *FT Weekend Magazine* for permission to reproduce parts of many of the columns again here.

A part of the chapter 'The Mysteries Within' appeared in an essay I wrote for the *London Review of Books*; many thanks to the *LRB* for permission to reproduce here.

Thank you to Peter Straus and Ursula Doyle, for believing in the book; and to Zoe Gullen, for helping me spell resuscitation.

A very big thank you to all the doctors, nurses, healthcare assistants, clinical support workers, pharmacists, physios, OTs, midwives, receptionists, medical students and GP trainees who have taught me, and who are still teaching me, how to be a doctor. Thanks to all the patients for putting up with me while I learn.

Thanks to Raj, for taking care of us all. I wish you didn't play the soundtrack to *Rocky III* so frequently, but I know your intentions are always good. Thanks to Hari and Sara, for bringing joy every day; to my parents, for their love, and for being so wise; and my brother Tom, for always letting me stay. To Sam and Sue Banerjee, for their endless generosity; and Ron, for understanding what it's like to live with Raj. Thank you to all the friends who have listened to me, and never let on they were bored, especially Gail Craig, Cari Kirby, Gail Lynch and Susie Renshaw. Thanks to Ian Jack and everyone at Granta from 1997 to 2003, who made it such a difficult place to leave.

Thanks in particular to my brother Jon, who is the hero of this book.

In memory of Alfie Harrison, 31.1.2010 – 29.3.2010; and Rachel Banerjee, 24.5.1985 – 15.8.2014.

18\2\22

PILLGWENLLY